Meetings and Moderation

Jochem Kießling-Sonntag

LEADS PRESS
An imprint of

B. Jain Publishers (P) Ltd.
An ISO 9001 : 2000 Certified Company
USA — Europe — India

MEETINGS AND MODERATION

First Indian Edition: 2010
1st Impression: 2010

All rights reserved. No part of this book may be reproduced, stored in a retrieval system or transmitted, in any form or by any means, mechanical, photocopying, recording or otherwise, without any prior written permission of the publisher.

© with the Author

Published by Kuldeep Jain for

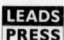

An imprint of
B. Jain Publishers (P) Ltd.
An ISO 9001 : 2000 certified Company
1921/10, Chuna Mandi, Paharganj, New Delhi 110 055 (INDIA)
Tel.: 91-11-4567 1000 • *Fax:* 91-11-4567 1010
Email: info@bjain.com • *Website:* **www.bjainbooks.com**

Printed in India by
J.J. Offset Printers

ISBN: 978-81-319-0854-9

Contents

Foreword vii

Part A Preparation

1 Slim & Trim Meetings 1

2 What We Can and Want to Achieve with the Meeting 7

2.1 The Framework: Limits and Leeway in Preparing the Subject Matter 7

2.2 Information Exchange, Searching for Solutions, Decision-Making – Central Types of Goals in Meetings 10

2.3 Formulate Aims in a Defined and Assessable Manner 12

2.4 Beyond Tough Goals: Additional Important Functions of Meetings 15
  Communication Styles 17

2.5 When One Should Forgo a Meeting 20

3 The Agenda 22

3.1 The Agenda as the Assignment Basis for an External Moderator 22

3.2 Components of the Agenda 23

3.3 The Process of Preparing the Agenda 26

3.4 From the Agenda to a Script for Moderation 26

3.5 The Form of the Invitation 29

4 Selecting the Group of Participants 30

5 Organisational Matters 33

5.1 Selection of the Meeting Location 33

5.2 Meeting Room Requirements 34
5.3 The Seating Arrangement 35

Part B Execution

1 Direction of the Course of the Meeting 39

1.1 The Introduction 39
1.2 Clarification of Topics, Objectives and Organisational Matters 41
1.3 Working on the Topics 43
1.4 Compilation of Results – Measures 45
1.5 The Conclusion 46

2 Meeting Direction as a Moderation Task 49

2.1 Giving the Floor 49
2.2 Posing Questions 51
2.3 Active Listening 55
2.4 Reformulating Statements, Introducing Compilations 56
2.5 Offer a Change of Focus 57
2.6 Reframing 58
2.7 Tactful Blocking 59
2.8 Flashlight Rounds 60

3 Provide Structure 62

3.1 Problem-Solving Procedure 62
3.2 Work Phases in Workshop Moderation 64

4 Moderation Techniques and Visualisations in Support of the Process 66

4.1 Media in Group Communication 66
    Presenting in front of an International Team 70
4.2 Work and Visualisation Techniques for Groups 72
4.3 Rules for Meetings 91

Contents

5 Roles and Posture of the Moderator 94

5.1 A Manager as Moderator 94
5.2 A Team Colleague of Equal Rank as the Moderator 95
   Individualism vs. Collectivism 96
5.3 An External Moderator to Guide the Process 97
5.4 The Neutral, Appreciative Posture of the Moderator 99

6 Guiding the Group Process 101

6.1 Four Levels of Group Communication 101
6.2 Moderation as Team Development 108

7 Dealing with Challenging Behaviour 112

8 Conflict Clarification 115

8.1 Signs of Conflict Dynamics – The Progression of
    Conflicts 115
8.2 Active Conflict Mediation 118

Part C Follow-Up

1 The Minutes 120

1.1 The Role of the Minutes Taker 120
1.2 Components of the Minutes 121
1.3 Minutes Standard and Form 122
1.4 Photo Minutes 122

2 Supporting Implementation 124

3 Personal Follow-Up Work of the Moderator 125

Bibliography 131

Foreword

Personal get-togethers in meetings continue to play a prominent role in the daily life of business. Communication consumes up to 90 percent of the working time of management personnel, and along with face-to-face dialogues and telephone calls, participating in meetings makes up the largest share of the communication tasks that have to be completed. This means that the ability to arrange meetings effectively and in a manner that is interpersonally satisfying is a prerequisite for professional success.

Aside from managing meetings, workshops are often the forum used for working out solutions. Building on the competence as a meetings supervisor, the moderator has numerous opportunities in workshops to provide support for the work of the respective group. (Even though the terminology in this book does not always refer specifically to male or female, both men and women are addressed equally throughout its pages.)

In this book, you will find the tools that you need for efficient meetings and solution-oriented moderating. We will focus initially on the preparation for meetings and workshops. Afterwards, we will concentrate on how you as the moderator can best promote the work of the group. And in conclusion, we will direct our attention to the question of how to follow up on meetings so that their results are put into practice. The appendix contains a questionnaire that you can use together with your team to analyse and further improve the meeting culture in your own working environment.

The internationalisation of business practice has resulted in a significant alignment or conformity of how meetings are conducted, particularly in the English-speaking and German-speaking world. An orientation on goals and structured procedure are priorities in both cultural territories. And in the German-speaking world, the realisation, long practised in English-speaking circles, has asserted itself that strongly-held positions should not be represented by "brushing off" the discussion partner, but rather by proceeding in a verbally respectful manner.

This book is intended to help you in meetings – also at the international level – to maintain an overview and to use your individual sovereignty to exercise a positive influence on the group and on the working process. With this in mind, I wish you good, sustainable and effective results for your meetings.

Jochem Kießling-Sonntag   Werther, Germany – Summer 2007

Part A Preparation

Meetings should not be stiff, artificial events; on the contrary, they should run as naturally as possible. And you should only use as many methodical and organisational tools as you genuinely need in order to reach the objectives of your meetings.

1 Slim & Trim Meetings

A Plea for Implicitness

Humans have always consulted with one another. The art of communicating with one another to come up with plans stretches back into antiquity. Indeed, in every culture the wise, the elders or the highest ranking persons in a community have met to discuss existential matters such as the food supply, dealing with deficiencies, war and peace, settling down or moving on, the sanctioning of individual members of the community in cases of unacceptable behaviour and many other important matters of cohabitation, with the ultimate aim of doing the right thing by their individual deities and traditions. To my knowledge, there were no flip charts or beamers in earlier times, and still many of the decisions made were correct and good; otherwise, the respective communities would not have been capable of surviving and developing into the societies of our time, which are extensively based on collective decision-making.

On the other side of the coin, there has always been and still exists today the world of power, of breaching the rules and of aggression that hinders, sabotages or uses violence to invalidate decision-making processes within a group. And of course, many mixed forms are evident in which the discourse is permeated with arguments, manipulation and the threat or exercise of instruments of power against the opposite party and in which the wrestling of these various powers then results in a consensus.

All of these processes are completely normal. Our ability to arrange meeting processes is one of our basic human tools, acquired from childhood onwards. So when we participate in a meeting, the first thing we use is our normal capability to communicate. In many cases, a discussion that develops naturally is sufficient for coming up with good solutions. In such cases, it is not necessary to apply special problem-solving techniques; corresponding structuring attempts might justifiably be perceived as awkward – and simultaneously as threatening, because the attempt to "stamp" an identity onto a discussion by applying a particular methodology to it could also be perceived as inappropriately dominant behaviour or an attempt at manipulation.

Since today's forms of cohabitation are much more complicated than in earlier times, with traditions fading and appreciably more innovative solutions having to be found for evermore surprising themes, discussions also require – especially in larger groups – evermore sophisticated meeting "tools". You will find all of these topics addressed extensively in this book.

Good meetings are subordinate to their purpose. Employee time is an increasingly costly commodity, with the result that the duration of meetings is correspondingly being reduced to the minimum. Individual preparation work on the part of the participants is obligatory and accelerates decision-making processes. The course of meetings is often heavily structured and the talk with one another direct, without much embellishment. And with the implementation of media tools as well, one can observe a trend towards concentration on the essential; simply put, it is easy to go overboard. For instance, beamer presentations displaying graphic finesse often create more distance than closeness; if such presentations are too elaborate, they are meanwhile frowned upon in some organisations as the expression of a lack of genuinely important tasks. For this reason, this wonderful technical possibility should not be overused, particularly in the framework of meetings.

> *Use the least possible amount of technical and methodical complexity and the greatest amount of time possible for mutual exchange.*

In practice, this can mean using flip charts instead of beamers, three charts instead of thirteen or a presentation of the five most important figures instead of a comprehensive depiction of a matrix with fifty-five figures. Additional information can be provided as supplemental background material. You can still use special methods when the subject matter requires it or when the team is not making progress with the usual procedure.

You may well see your meetings increase in efficiency and generally be more pleasant all around if you use the time saved by forgoing unnecessary methodical effort instead for more intensive mutual listening on the part of the participants, as well as perhaps also for more breaks to think about what has been said. The most relaxed, natural supervision of a meeting possible gives all its participants a feeling of security, stabilises self-confidence in expressing one's own interests, forms the foundation for an atmosphere of appreciation and makes it easier to reach sustainable results. In contrast, a meeting overly characterised by the application of methodology and the implementation of multi-media often diverts the gaze from what is important; not infrequently, it also conceals the personal excessive demands of the meeting director and prevents the creation of the ultimately important pleasant working environment.

Good meetings are already a part of the day-to-day in many organisations. Teamwork, interdisciplinary projects, planning and coordinative tasks require regular meetings with those involved. Meetings results are sometimes of great importance, as meetings represent the forum where the ground is laid for decisions with long-term consequences. People get together in a no-frills manner in a conference room or larger office. There may be coffee and soft drinks on hand. The procedure is governed by standardised formulae and the unwritten rules of the internal meeting culture. Some considerations are documented on a flip chart. All of the participants are familiar with the duration and style of the moderation. One can address the contents and the desired objectives. Work results are recorded in brief phrases and quickly made available to all the participants and all those affected. The only arrangements made are those that can be realistically realised and that facilitate the progress of the team.

In other organisations on the other hand, meetings as a management instrument are not (yet) such an integral part of the daily agenda. In such organisations, it is often only the management staff that uses regular meetings as a forum for the exchange of information. In the operative course of business, much is decided alone by the owner, the managing director or the respective management person invested with such responsibility. Employees would like to implement more of their knowledge and experience in the work, and they would also like to receive more information on a regular basis about current developments, but their involvement is not called upon. In an organisation like this, anyone who sends an invitation to a meeting, perhaps even with an agenda attached, can come across as slightly suspect: Does the formal manner of procedure translate into bad news? Does the boss want to introduce a new way of doing things in which he or she is relying on documenting things as a means of control?

A look at these "opposite poles" of organisations with and without an emphasis on meetings makes it clear that it is the "dosage" that counts! The more know-how regarding "effective meeting management" that is already anchored within the organisation and the more of its people who know their way around professionally conducted meetings, the easier it is to implement new meetings techniques. In contrast, in an organisation where meetings are the exception rather than the rule, one should initially start with small steps; for instance, asking sometime during the beginning of the meeting how long it will last, which topics should be discussed and in what order. For some organisations, even complying with a schedule is already a big step.

Meetings are regarded as successful when they result in attaining firm objectives and solving problems.

The output is the decisive issue. It is easy to establish the degree to which tangible results emerge from the arranged meetings and the extent to which these are then implemented in practice. Results that are prepared and implemented together are a good indicator that the personal chemistry in the team is right, because relationship problems in a team are almost always reflected in the quality of the results. The typical behavioural patterns indicating disruptions within the group and negatively affecting the results of the meeting are easy to spot: Endless discussions about matters of secondary importance, "postpone-itis", long monologues, self-justifications or killer phrases like, *"But we've always done it that way."*

But when the participants take the initiative, provide recommendations for action, when they also demonstrate respect for opposing views, take on assignments and are capable of managing the discussion process for longer periods without the help of the moderator, then your team is on the right track, not just in regard to the skills needed for the job, but also interpersonally.

In the following pages, you will repeatedly come across the designations, "Meeting" and "Workshop". Here is a brief distinction between the two:

Meeting	Workshop
• Generally a small number of participants: 2–10 persons	• Generally a medium-sized number of participants: 5–30 persons
• The objective is the exchange of information, the coordination/delegation of tasks	• The objectives are clarifying problems, brainstorming, implementation planning and, to some extent also, advanced training – the theme is often (still) less specific
• Meetings frequently take place more regularly, for example, a weekly team meeting	• Workshops are usually conducted as needed; generally not on a cyclical basis
• The duration can consist of a few minutes to a full-day meeting	• The duration can consist of a few hours to several days

2 What We Can and Want to Achieve with the Meeting

Goal Setting

Insufficient goal setting and the failure to provide important information on what kind of work leeway the group possesses are reasons why meetings leave their participants unsatisfied. Formulating objectives clearly is one of the most important success factors for effective, motivating meetings.

2.1 The Framework: Limits and Leeway in Preparing the Subject Matter

You should consider limits and leeway in meetings above all when topics are up for discussion that are highly emotional or for which the attendant work is likely to lead to grave consequences in the company. It is essential in such cases to be acutely aware of what is negotiable in the meeting and what is not.

Here is a brief example as an introduction: *A Sales Department manager has called a meeting on the subject of "Process Optimisation in Order Entry". She briefly introduces the topic and in turn the affected employees present at the meeting begin collecting ideas on reducing mistakes, on cooperation with the Field Sales Staff and on simplifying the processes. Over the next 30 minutes, the employees – unhindered by the manager – make a wealth of suggestions, and some resentment emerges: Unclear departmental responsibilities or orders incorrectly documented by Field Sales Staff employees are a source of irritation. The manager abruptly ends the discussion. She presents a few charts that, in her view, outline the problem situation and additionally already precisely define countermeasures, for example, that describe changes in customer allocations. The manager has already made the decision to implement these measures; she now specifically describes the consequences that the changes will have for the employees. There is no room for the recommended changes the employees have just made. The employees feel completely snubbed.*

The first question this situation raises is whether it was at all wise of the manager to have already decided upon the measures to be undertaken even before the meeting. But perhaps she was herself acting on instructions whereby she was forced to present the group with a decision that had already been made. It is possible that personnel changes had already been decided at a higher level that will bring a restructuring of the department in their wake, and for which the manager is not permitted to pass on all of the information about the changes in its entirety. In any case, it would have made sense to openly inform the team at the start of the meeting what the topic of discussion is, which assessments can already be discussed, which questions are still unresolved and which matters can be clarified among one another.

> *Information about the framework in which work can be conducted together has the highest priority, and it should be provided at the start of the meeting or at the respective point on the agenda.*

Meetings take place in the interactive space between decisions that have already been made and the latitudes that can still be flexibly used. With important matters, the framework in which a group has leeway in the processing of the topic should without exception be established prior to the meeting or agreed upon with the decision-maker(s) / principal party or parties.

What We Can Achieve with the Meeting

If the meeting is being directed by a higher ranking individual, then it is their job to communicate this framework clearly. If an external moderator is appointed or an employee of lower or equal rank is conducting the meeting, then this framework should be precisely agreed upon with that person.

The varying degrees of prior establishment and the resulting latitudes are depicted below in the renowned "Delegation Continuum".

I have decided:	and you are invited to discuss with me:	Example
Nothing	Whether something should be done	*Meeting about whether it makes sense to initiate a project on the subject of "Process Optimisation" within the department*
That something should be done	What should be done	*Meeting about how this kind of project could be arranged*
What should be done	When, how, where and by whom it should be done	*Meeting about how measures that have already been decided can be implemented*
When, how, where and by whom it should be done	The reasons for my decision	*An open discussion with the team about why, in a crisis situation, certain measures had to be decided without feedback from the team*
Everything	Nothing; I just want to hear what the associated consequences are for you	*Questioning of the team focusing on how it aims to guarantee the implementation of measures that have been decided and announced*
Everything	Nothing	*The team receives instructions regarding procedural changes that have been decided; these can also be supplied in writing*

Ill. 1: The Delegation Continuum (according to Schwarz in Antons 2000, p. 174, supplemented with examples)

Certainly, the type of authoritarian manner depicted in the final line is hardly to be recommended. Nevertheless, it is important, for example in the case of strict instructions from top management, to be careful with hasty judgments: Even restricted latitudes will often be accepted by the group if sound reasons are given for the procedure and the director of the meeting acts in a way that is fair and transparent.

2.2 Information Exchange, Searching for Solutions, Decision-Making – Central Types of Goals in Meetings

In meetings and conferences, the aim in most cases is the processing of facts. This distinguishes meetings somewhat from team development workshops and many employee discussions that can also be focused on the work relationship as a topic of discussion. Naturally, a meeting on facts is also always embedded in a specific work climate; but in the day-to-day exercise of meetings, addressing sensibilities and emotional relationships is rarely among the primary objects of discussion.

The exchange of information, the search for solutions and decision-making are the three central aims in meetings.

The Information Exchange Meeting

An information meeting is often a routine get-together, for instance, the "monthly management meeting": The executive managers of a company provide each other with information regarding key data and trends so that all of the important decision-makers in the firm are up to date and are able to register deviations in planning data early on.

A meeting in which managers inform their teams about short-term and mid-term plans and decisions also falls under this category of meeting: In many cases, after receiving the information, the employees then receive straightforward instructions.

The participants are invited to provide their appraisals. Questions regarding the understanding of the topic or instructions can be clarified. In contrast, fundamental discussions questioning decisions that have already been made or that are aimed at the mutual adoption of measures are not appropriate here.

However, the character of the meeting can change if the manager is confronted with facts that make planned directives unfeasible (for example, the sudden illness of an employee): In such a case, the information meeting can now become a solution-seeking meeting under certain circumstances.

The Solution Search Meeting

The majority of meetings fall under this category. For example, this applies to project meetings and workshops in which often questions and objectives that are ambiguous are developed and steps for implementation are given preliminary consideration. Creativity is the thing most in demand at meetings in search of solutions, but adeptness in one's dealings with the group of participants is also called for, because the object is not just to produce as many ideas as possible, but also to come up with solutions that will receive the broadest positive response in the group. The meeting director's skills in guiding the social process of the group face their greatest challenge here.

The Decision-Making Meeting

Decision-making is often exercised in formal conferences with a high-ranking group of participants. Possible solutions have generally been prepared in advance. Now the question arises, *"Which solution alternative do we pick?"* Or, if there is only one new recommendation for action, *"Do we do it or don't we?"* Decision-making meetings are often chaired by the highest-ranking participant.

Many meetings are mixed forms of the three basic types described above. Here is an example: For one of the agenda items in a meeting, there is only one progress report from a team member with no necessity for a decision and action; in conclusion, a solution for a difficult operative question is sought and finally, the entire team reaches a budget decision regarding a completely separate matter.

Information Acquisition, Solution Search and Decision-Making as Three Steps to Problem-Solving

Many problem-solving cycles can often be designed sensibly as a chronological progression of these three work-related steps: Information acquisition, the search for a solution and decision-making. Particularly in the case of complex topics with significant consequences, it often makes sense to redress the procedure. Especially in the early work phases where the priority is analysis of the situation, this can ease the performance pressure that so frequently leads to blind action for its own sake, but not to sustainable measures. Solutions reached too quickly often lead precisely to unforeseen side effects as well as to emotional resistance on the part of the people involved, since they feel insufficiently included in the problem-solving process.

2.3 Formulate Aims in a Defined and Assessable Manner

Clearly formulated aims are the best tool for being able to evaluate the success of your meeting. As the person in charge, you should already clarify for yourself in the planning exactly what it is you want to achieve with the meeting. If possible though, you should not prescribe the aims of the meeting for the participants, but instead agree them in the introductory phase together with the group.

So the sequence looks like this:
1. Prepare a goal recommendation for the meeting in the planning.
2. Recommend the prepared goal to the group of participants at the beginning of the meeting.
3. Get the acceptance or response of the group on the matter. For this, you can use formulations such as: *"In today's meeting, we should do the preliminary planning for the next six weeks. What do you all think about that?"*

If the group of participants does not agree, you can modify the recommendation or ask the group to make an alternative suggestion.

Mutual clarification of sensible meeting aims takes a little time, but you usually win it back in the end since you now have everyone "pulling in the same direction".

The Benefit of Goals in Conducting Meetings
The orientation on firm goals brings a series of benefits for you and the participants:
- Attention is directed toward results right from the start; discussions are subsequently more focused
- Agreed-upon meeting goals take the full weight of the load off the moderator, since the group can direct itself better on the basis of the clearly defined goals
- The work priorities are fully visible for everyone; this helps everyone to concentrate on what's important in the meeting
- Success can be directly verified on the basis of goals

- Participants work harder for a goal that they have helped to formulate themselves than for one that has been assigned to them by someone else
- It is fun reaching goals! Goals increase motivation

The SMART Formula for Formulating Goals

With the help of goals, visions for the future become visible and communicable. The precise description of what everyone wants to achieve together prevents misunderstandings in regard to the quality of the anticipated results.

> *The SMART-Formula has proven itself to be practicable for the formulation of goals, and according to it, goals are correctly and sensibly formulated when they meet the following criteria:*

S = Specific: Precise description of the desired condition, comprehensible formulation

M = Measurable: Designation of criteria as the basis for assessing success

A = Active influence: Goal is in the group's sphere of responsibility

R = Relevant: Decisive for the success of the company, the project, the workgroup

T = Time-phased: Designation of the point in time by which the goal is to be reached

Example:
Goal – Superordinated context: *The goal to be achieved is an increase in sales of Product XY by 15 % within the next twelve months.* The group affected consists of the presiding Regional Directors for the sale of the product and the marketing employees for the product, enabling group attainment of the goal to be

actively influenced by the group. The criteria regarding the description, measurability, relevance and time-phasing of the goal are equally fulfilled.

Therefore, work in the meeting is focused on defined subordinate parts of the goal. This is demonstrated in the following examples.

- Possible Meeting Goal – Information Acquisition Phase:
  Compilation of all internal and external influence factors currently detracting from sales of Product XY; development of future scenarios on the basis of market forecasts
- Possible Meeting Goal – Solution Search Phase:
  Collection and prioritisation of possible activities with which sales can be increased to meet the goal
- Possible Meeting Goal – Decision-Making Phase:
  Preparation of the decision for sales-boosting Sales Department activities within the next twelve months on the basis of the recommendations developed by the workgroup

2.4 Beyond Tough Goals: Additional Important Functions of Meetings

People want to experience themselves as a part of their reference group and to have the opportunity within this group to express their interests and needs. We spend a large part of our lives in the workplace, making the team in which we work an important social place for us.

Already in your planning for the meeting, you should keep an eye on how much room you want to leave for informal interaction and the needs that the participants bring into the meeting in their respective roles within the group.

Maintaining Contacts

The participants who assemble for a meeting often have little opportunity in their professional day-to-day to talk with one another. Prior to the start of the actual meeting, one sees the participants standing together engaged in lively conversation. Some have become friends through working together and are talking about their private lives, while others exchange experiences and news, and still others are coordinating final details. The personal contact that meetings enable is irreplaceable – even through telephone or video conferences.

Tips for preparing informal encounter opportunities in the meeting

- *Rule of thumb: The more infrequently the participants meet and the more important the work of the group is, the more time you should plan for informal encounter opportunities.*
- *Set up the meeting room early and provide beverages before the meeting starts so that the participants can already assemble casually in a pleasant atmosphere.*
- *If time is short and you want to avoid the informal encounter spilling over into the appointed meeting time, start with the meeting punctually and tell the participants when they will have time to meet informally afterwards (for example, at lunch).*
- *If the group only assembles on an infrequent basis, it is recommended to arrange an "extracurricular activity" (for instance, a dinner together outside of work). This upgrades the value of the meeting and has a motivating effect.*

Promote the Group Process

Workgroups can achieve good results when their members can interact with one another in a trusting atmosphere free of fear. It is important that the group sticks together as a matter of principle and that everyone knows or can find their place within the group.

Communication Styles

What do you think is happening here?

The German marketing manager of a major car producer was finding it increasingly difficult to work in Japan. In meetings the Japanese colleagues hardly ever said anything. When they were asked if they agreed to his suggestions they always said yes, but they didn't do anything to follow up the ideas. The only time they opened up was in a bar in the evening but that was getting stressful as they seemed to expect him to go out with them regularly.

According to Edward T. Hall (1976), in high context cultures, like Japan, meaning does not always have to be put into words. Non-verbal clues are important as is the context in which the situation takes place. Even the meaning of words can depend on the context: "yes" can mean anything from "I agree", to "I am listening" to "no". Relationship building is important in high context cultures and there is an emphasis on getting to know the business partner. In low context cultures (like Germany and the USA) meaning is made explicit and put into words. These cultures tend to be task-centred rather than relationship-centred.

The diagrams show Hall's concept and a possible positioning of some national cultures on the scale low – high context.

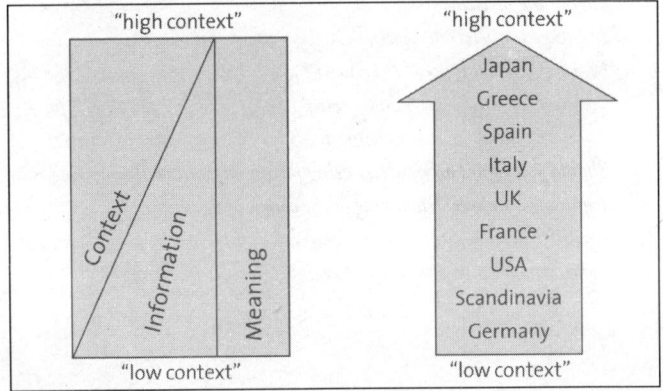

Open questions must be cleared up so that the group's attention is not distracted from the actual topic of discussion any longer than necessary.

The following consideration questions can help you to be clear about the team's situation in advance. (cp. Part B, Chapter 6–8)

Consideration questions for promoting group processes within the meeting

- *Are new participants going to be on hand, requiring a round of introductions at the beginning of the meeting?*
- *Are the responsibilities of the participants clear, or are there questions or ambiguities that need to be answered?*
- *Do all of the members feel comfortable in their current roles, or should you count on expressions of dissatisfaction that should be brought up for discussion?*
- *Are there agenda items that are inherently highly emotional since participants are significantly affected by them on a personal level?*
- *Are there persons who explicitly oppose plans that should be mentioned during the meeting?*
- *Are there conflicts over and above the context of the meeting that are begging to be addressed? Does working on these conflicts make sense in the meeting, or should another setting be sought for that subject (for instance, a personal discussion with the person or persons in question)?*
- *Should you figure on rivalries being fought out within the meeting, requiring a stricter structuring of the course of discussion?*
- *Are there devalued persons or scapegoats in the team requiring above all that the moderator proceed in way that promotes integration?*

Increasing Motivation

Meetings provide you with an ideal forum to promote employee motivation. By emphasising successes that have been achieved together in the meeting, by developing interesting future scenarios and above all, through active work together on solutions to problems, you, as the meeting director, can positively influence the performance motivation of the participants.

Motivation-promoting activities in meetings

- *Promptly give specific, honest feedback on achieved results (for example, sales development); transparency stimulates and promotes performance motivation.*
- *Talk about successes achieved together, celebrate them! Success attracts success. And positive results increase identification with the team.*
- *Be reserved with the use of material rewards as an enticement. The motivating effect dissipates quickly and the group members can easily be misled into avoiding long-term tasks in favour of short-term activities.*
- *Highlight the group's strengths. This stabilises the positive conduct demonstrated (for example, deadline punctuality, flexibility, inventiveness).*
- *Depict even difficult situations (for instance, reduced market share, declining profits) as changeable, because we only make an effort when we perceive the situation in question as one that is capable of being influenced.*
- *Demonstrate that the consequences your work together in the meeting can have are worthwhile for everyone, because we only make an effort for goals that have a positive character.*
- *Describe the goals of the work together in simple, specific and measurable (cp. Part A, Chapter 2.3) terms, because only in this way can they be a good beacon for the mutual activities.*

- *Make sure that all of the activities in the meeting are in accord with basic human needs:*
  - *Security (for instance, job security)*
  - *Autonomy (for instance, that completion of the tasks foresees latitudes)*
  - *Experiencing one's own competence (no chronic excessive demands; feeling fundamentally capable of meeting the demands)*
  - *Feeling integrated within the group*
- *Switch off factors that diminish motivation (for instance, a fanaticism for order, lone decision-making, personal criticism of individuals in the presence of the group, failing to pass on or insufficiently passing on information).*

2.5 When One Should Forgo a Meeting

A meeting is not always necessary to reach a certain working goal. Managers and employees often feel detained from more important duties by meetings, and the antipathy toward the ever-present "meeting tourism" then also shows its ugly head in genuinely important meetings.

The invited participants have a high level of sensitivity regarding the amount of time expected of them for a meeting. Above all, it is counterproductive to call a meeting when sensitive topics are not yet ripe for being made public.

The following brief checklist provides a few clues for when you should refrain from holding a meeting:

- The assignment for the team is not (yet) sufficiently clarified, leaving a lack of clearly defined questions for discussion
- The project and meeting objectives are still unclear
- Participants important for the subject of the meeting cannot attend

What We Can Achieve with the Meeting

- The available information is insufficient for properly preparing and conducting the conference
- The preparation time is too short
- Confidential topics are on the agenda that should not be presented to the entire group
- The topics in question are neither important nor urgent
- The topics in question are indeed important, but current events or tasks with top priority take up so much of the participants' energy that holding a conference at this time would probably be of no benefit
- Deep conflicts have arisen between participants that block constructive cooperation and have to be settled first
- There are more efficient ways to deal with the tasks at hand (for example, direct delegation of tasks to individual employees)

3 The Agenda

Meetings without an agenda regularly lead to becoming bogged down which results in the available time being insufficient. One touches somehow on important topics, planned topics are perhaps discussed at random; after a while, the lack of structure and overview often leads to a deterioration of the overall mood in the group. Afterwards one thinks, *"I could have done without that meeting"*. So the rule is:

> *The agenda is the single most important orientation tool for the meeting.*

The agenda puts the topics for the meeting into a logical order. The agenda provides a basis for estimating how much time is available for each of the individual items. And last but not least, it makes it possible to monitor success: Which items could be finalised? What could not be addressed due to a lack of time?

Of course, it takes time to create an agenda and to agree on it with the participants prior to a meeting, but the effort is generally rewarded in the form of more efficient progress and a much more stable, pleasant working process.

In exceptional cases, in a crisis situation for instance, preparing an agenda is not possible. The director of the meeting should then create the agenda at the beginning of the meeting together with the participants and document it on a flip chart for all to see.

3.1 The Agenda as the Assignment Basis for an External Moderator

If the meeting is going to be conducted by an external moderator, then the agenda is one if not the central basis for his or her assignment. Often, agreement on the agenda between the contractor – e.g. a manager – and the moderator is the first step to successfully directing the workgroup, particularly in the case of work on difficult subjects.

Careful clarification of the meeting items and their sequence helps ...

- to find out what can be discussed and which topics should be left out
- to formulate clear objectives for the moderating job
- to avoid overly-ambitious objectives
- to find out where information is missing that should be provided to the participants prior to the event
- to realistically set the timeframes for the meeting
- to establish criteria for who should be invited
- to determine which items are likely to encounter resistance

Ambiguities on the part of the contractor are often based in the fact that he or she has not yet given these aspects enough consideration. A lack of experience frequently makes it impossible for him or her to create a meeting plan that stands up even in the midst of a crisis and still allows the greatest possible prospects for success.

As an external moderator, a carefully planned agenda also gives you an additional psychological advantage: You can feel well-prepared since you have planned what's "plan-able" and have been able to develop a sense of which unknown factors exist. This allows you to meet surprises more calmly. If the agenda cannot be worked through as planned, you can still change it in consultation with the group and the contractor during the course of the meeting.

3.2 Components of the Agenda

Indispensable elements of the agenda:

- The date (day and time) and the meeting location
- The topics to be discussed and their sequence

In preparing for routine meetings, this information is often enough.

Depending on the importance of the topics, the composition of the group and the corporate culture, you can also include additional elements in the agenda:
- A list of the invited participants
- The person calling the meeting or the host
- The moderator
- The person responsible for the minutes
- Preparation assignments for the participants and responsibilities for the topics
- The aims of the meeting for each of the agenda items
- The starting time for beginning work on each of the agenda items

When creating the agenda you should observe the following aspects:
- Keep the agenda brief and to the point:
  - not too many meeting items
  - agenda items in heading form
- Number the agenda items
- Pay attention to a sensible sequence of the topics – possibilities:
  - Timing logic (the most urgent first)
  - According to priorities (the most important first)
  - Starting with routine topics (to warm up the group)
  - Starting with uncontroversial topics (reinforce positive atmosphere)
- Adapt the allotted time for the individual topics according to the importance and complexity of the topics
- Err on the side of setting aside too much time rather than too little – everyone likes finishing early, but running over is usually irritating

The Agenda

Monthly Team Meeting of the Sales Department Employees

Date:	Oct. 27, 2007
Time:	9:00 a.m.–11:00 a.m.
Location:	Room 7.21
Called by:	F. Hackert
Moderation:	A. Beltermann
Minutes:	P. Orschel
Participants:	O. Dinkelborg, H. Venker, M. Nettels, H. Janssen, E. Glombitza, P. Kruschka
Enclosed material:	– –
Please prepare:	Ideas for regional customer acquisition

October 4th, 2007

Dear colleagues,

I would herewith like to invite you to the next Team Meeting. I look forward to a lively, constructive discussion with all of you!

Best regards,
F. Hackert

Agenda

Topic	Objective	Responsible Party	Time
1. Opening	– –	F. Hackert	9:00
2. Realisation of the results of the meeting on Sept. 20, 2007	Information	A. Beltermann	9:10
3. 3rd Quarter sales results, introduction of new products, new brochure material	Information	F. Hackert	9:30
4. Introduction of ideas for regional customer acquisition	Information/ Decision	All Sales Dept. employees	9:50
5. Recommendations for new product ideas	Brainstorming	A. Beltermann	10:15
6. Miscellaneous	– –	A. Beltermann	10:45
7. Conclusion	– –	F. Hackert	10:55

Ill. 2: Sample agenda

3.3 The Process of Preparing the Agenda

You should prepare the agenda early and send it to the participants. This improves the quality of the results and the willingness of the participants to cooperate. In contrast, surprising negatively tinged topics, unfounded last-minute programme changes or holding back important information in advance fosters resistance.

So include your team early on in creating the agenda.

You can proceed as follows in creating an agenda:
1. Agree upon a date and time for the meeting.
2. Compile relevant agenda items and formulate a sensible meeting aim for each topic.
3. Put the meeting topics into a preliminary order.
4. Send the agenda draft to the participants and request their response and possible amendments
5. Integrate the amendment recommendations into the agenda.
6. If need be, delegate tasks for preparing important information for the meeting.
7. Send the final agenda and important information to the participants.

3.4 From the Agenda to a Script for Moderation

For very important meetings or when you want to implement methodically complex working steps in a meeting, a customary agenda is often insufficient for the advance planning of the

The Agenda

event. In such cases, you can create a "script". The degree to which it is detailed can vary greatly.

Elements of the script can include:
- Scheduled times for the working steps, including breaks
- Agenda items in the order that they should be worked on
- A detailed description of each of the working steps
- Objectives of each of the working steps
- Methods with which to approach them
- Required media
- Appointment of a person primarily responsible for dealing with each step

The script is your personal procedure documentation which you can also use as the basis for agreeing on the working steps with other persons who are taking on a part in the meeting.

However, it is not necessary and usually also not advisable to issue the script to all of the meeting participants. If you did, you would heavily limit your options as the moderator and would hardly be in a position to work your way out of the situation. The participants would easily adopt a mild sort of "monitoring posture" toward you (*"Is the moderator doing everything as it's described in the script?"*). The agenda and info materials are generally sufficient as orientation tools for the participants. As the moderator, you should maintain the flexibility to deviate from your script if necessary.

Here is an excerpt from a fairly comprehensive meeting script:

Time	Topic	Working step	Objective of the working step	Method	Media	Responsible party
...	...	...	...	...	...	...
10:15	Recommendations for new product ideas	Introduction to the agenda item	Depicting the great significance of new products for the success of the company	Briefly familiarising		F. Hackert
10:20		Product presentation	Informing the participants of their possibilities for influencing the matter – Motivating	Presentation of Product XY, which came out of an earlier creativity meeting	Demonstration of Product XY	F. Hackert
10:25		Presentation of the brainstorming rules	Conveying the importance of complying with the rules	Brief input	Depiction of the rules on a flip chart	A. Beltermann
10:30		Conducting the brainstorming	Generating ideas	Brainstorming in the plenum	Noting the ideas on the flip chart	A. Beltermann
...			...	...	...	...

Ill. 3: Excerpt from a meeting script

3.5 The Form of the Invitation

For routine meetings, an informal or very brief invitation to the group of participants is often adequate. If a larger group is assembling that meets, let's say, once a year within the framework of an important conference, then it is recommended to send the participants a formal written invitation. In this way, you stress the importance of the meeting and, additionally, you give the participants the opportunity early on to integrate the meeting into their plans.

Recipient   *October 15th, 2007*

Dear Ms ... / Mr ...,

At this early stage, we would already like to invite you to attend our annual Executive Management Conference, to be held on December 15th & 16th, 2007 at Country Hotel X, near Y. We will send you arrivals information and the exact conference schedule around four weeks prior to the event.

As is customary every year, on the first day you will receive comprehensive information on current business developments and the plans for the upcoming year. On the second day, we will then have the opportunity for an intensive discussion covering the experiences of the participants under the direction of an external moderator. Please keep this date free for this important meeting!

On the evening of December 15th, you are cordially invited to our Christmas celebration.

We have already pre-booked a single room for you in the hotel for the evening of December 15th. Please confirm your participation within the next two weeks and let us know when you would like to arrive on December 14th so that we can make a corresponding reservation for you. Ms Z. (Tel.: ...) is available to help with any organisational questions you might have.

We look forward to an intensive working meeting and a festive close to the year!

Best regards

Ill. 4: Sample of a preliminary invitation

4 Selecting the Group of Participants

Who should be invited to the meeting?

It is impossible to establish an "ideal" group size for a meeting. If the meeting has a solely informative character, then there are no limitations. If, however, the object is to work together intensively developing creative solutions, then a small group consisting of a maximum of ten persons is certainly more capable of working than, for instance, a group of fifteen or more persons.

For situations with a schedule stretching over several hours involving larger groups, the formation of sub-groups is recommended who conduct work simultaneously during the meeting on partial aspects of the subject matter. On the other hand, for solution-oriented work, a group should also not be too small. Two or three persons, particularly when they know each other well, can tend to begin repeatedly falling back on approaches that have already been aired when looking for solutions.

For some meetings and conferences, the number of participants is prescribed by the organisational framework: **All of the team members participate in the team meeting; all of the shareholders participate in the shareholder's General Meeting.** To exclude someone in such cases would either be formally impermissible or at least highly insulting to the uninvited colleagues. In other types of meetings, the determination of the group of participants can be arranged more flexibly, for example in workshops with (as yet) less defined topics and aims, or meetings on starting up projects.

You should observe the following aspects in selecting the participants:

- **The technical skills of the participant**

Selecting the Group of Participants

- The decision-making power of the invited party
- The creativity of the participant
- "Political" factors (e.g. the invitation of opinion leaders)
- Group-dynamic aspects
  - The formation of a group with the greatest possible degree of diversity for a discussion covering the greatest possible number of angles
  - The invitation of a group with a great sense of affiliation in order to guarantee intensive cooperation

Tips for a sensible selection of meeting participants

- *Each participant should have an important function in relation to the objective of the meeting.*
- *Each participant should be equipped with the competence necessary to be able to contribute constructively.*
- *All of the technical or specialist skills essential for the solution of the problems on the agenda should be represented within the group of participants.*
- *Persons who are important for building trust within the group should be included in the invitations.*
- *Persons appointed with coordinative tasks – for example, in interdepartmental collaborations – should be included in the invitations.*
- *All of the parties invited should be prepared to assume assignments and responsibility in the problem-solving.*
- *When you have the impression that some persons want to participate in the planned meetings solely for reasons of prestige, you can introduce two types of meetings:*
  - *Meetings in which you genuinely conduct work on your topics with a small group of participants and*

- *Regular informational and decision-making meetings held at less frequent intervals in which you inform important persons from your organisation about the progress of the work and make recommendations for decisions.*

- When you have the impression that some of the meeting participants are making no significant contribution to finding solutions, then make sure that each participant receives an assignment with a deadline at the end of the conference. In this way, you increase the binding character of the meeting.

- *For important topics perhaps featuring less specific aims initially (e.g. "Improving the Work Atmosphere" or "Ideas for New Products"), you can first define the group of participants in larger terms and then invite participants more selectively in subsequent meetings.*

- The same applies when the object is to reach broad consensus: It is better to invite too many individuals in the first step than to risk creating resistance by "passing" on certain persons.

- *If the meeting is to be kept small, give the uninvited persons the assurance that they are not missing out on anything important. Arrange to send them the minutes of the meeting or to have an information meeting to inform them of the results of the smaller meeting.*

- In regularly-held work meetings with complex subject matter, it is not necessary to have all of the persons involved in the process present at the same time. For certain topics, you can invite the necessary dialogue partners who are then involved in the discussion only for the time that the agenda items relevant to their work are addressed.

5 Organisational Matters

The organisational effort required for meetings depends significantly on the number of participants and the choice of the meeting location. External events in rented conference rooms with a large group of participants require a great deal more logistical consideration than a lean internal meeting.

5.1 Selection of the Meeting Location

Possible alternatives consist of:

- The manager's office
  - Documentation is readily accessible
  - Emphasises the hierarchical context of the meeting
  - Disruptions by other employees and phone calls are often unavoidable

- An Employee's Office
  - Raises the profile of the employee
  - Could be a tight fit if the office is small
  - Disruptions from daily business possible

- Conference Room on Company Premises
  - "Neutral territory"
  - Media facilities usually on hand
  - Disruptions from other workers are often difficult to avoid
  - Reservation necessary

- External Meeting Location – e.g. Hotel
  - Rooms can be reserved in all sizes and equipment variations
  - Disruptions are eliminated
  - Raises the profile of the entire process (for example, "Conference")

- Possibilities include meeting, fringe programme, events, relaxation
- Increased organisational effort
- Increased expenses

5.2 Meeting Room Requirements

The characteristics of the room play a decisive role in influencing the quality of the communication.

Meeting room features that enhance communication are:

- Sufficient room space (Guideline: approximately 4 to 5 square metres per participant)
- Ideally daylight, but if possible no glare from direct sunlight
- Comfortable room proportions (preferably a rectangular format instead of a "long tube")
- Good ventilation, adequate heating, quiet air conditioning
- Good acoustics (no heavy reverberation)
- For large-scale events: microphone/P.A. system
- The possibility of darkening the room for presentations and projections
- Comfortable seating
- The possibility of attaching documentation on the working process (e.g. flip chart sheets) to the wall
- Media such as flip charts, pinboards, beamers, overhead projectors, screen available with no technical problems
- If necessary, having adjacent rooms for group work
- No external sources of disruption (for instance, building sites)

The larger the group of participants, the more important the meeting and the longer the duration of the conference, the more important it is that as many of the criteria specified above are fulfilled.

Organisational Matters

5.3 The Seating Arrangement

Seating should be arranged so that all of the participants have good visibility and can communicate with one another without any acoustic problems.

> *Additionally, the seating arrangement is often of symbolic importance.*

This is principally in regard to the visual expression of hierarchical functions or the conscious waiver of such. A typical example of a seating arrangement that emphasises the corresponding hierarchy would be putting the chairperson at the head of a long conference table. A well-known example of a seating arrangement that expresses the equality of the participants is the "round table".

A Round Table
All participants can see one another equally well. The seating arrangement symbolises the desire for cooperation and equality.

B Rectangular Seating Arrangement
This seating arrangement also emphasises a cooperative atmosphere. Nevertheless, the participants seated next to the director are not easily perceived by him or her. When a rectangular table is specified, other predestined participants can sit next to the Meeting Director, for example, a manager or topical expert.

C Large Rectangle for Assemblies and Conferences
Corresponds with Example B, only with a larger number of participants. If the arrangement of the tables were formed in a circle, the participants would be able to see each other even better.

D U-Shape for Events with Speakers

Events with a mid-sized number of participants (from approximately 10 to 30) are very frequently conducted in this seating arrangement – in particular advanced training events of a lecture-type nature.

Here (see sketch, Ill. 5) there is a seat next to the director for a second lecturer or the host.

E Circled Seating for Workshops

Circled seating has become a sort of standard in participant-active solution-seeking work. The director sits at the edge so that he or she can easily "take the stage" to speak, lead discussions or visualise work results. The dashes in the sketch symbolise media such as pinboards or flip charts, easily visible for all present. The equality of the participants is emphasised. It is easy to approach the front from every position. The easy access for everyone to the media and the space for physical activity positively influence the creativity of the participants. The disadvantage of this seating arrangement is the lack of space for storing work materials. Circled seating can also be created with larger numbers of participants; in some situations, a number of seating rows can be arranged one after the other in semi-circles. In events where media facilities play a lesser role, the semi-circle can also be replaced by a full circle without tables. The closed circle reinforces the group's cohesion even more than a semi-circle.

F Arrangement of Small Groups in the Room

In large rooms, smaller groups can retire to a corner with a pinboard or a flip chart. Work materials (pens & pencils, moderation cards, pins) and soft drinks should be provided at tables along the walls in sufficient quantity. After completion of

Organisational Matters

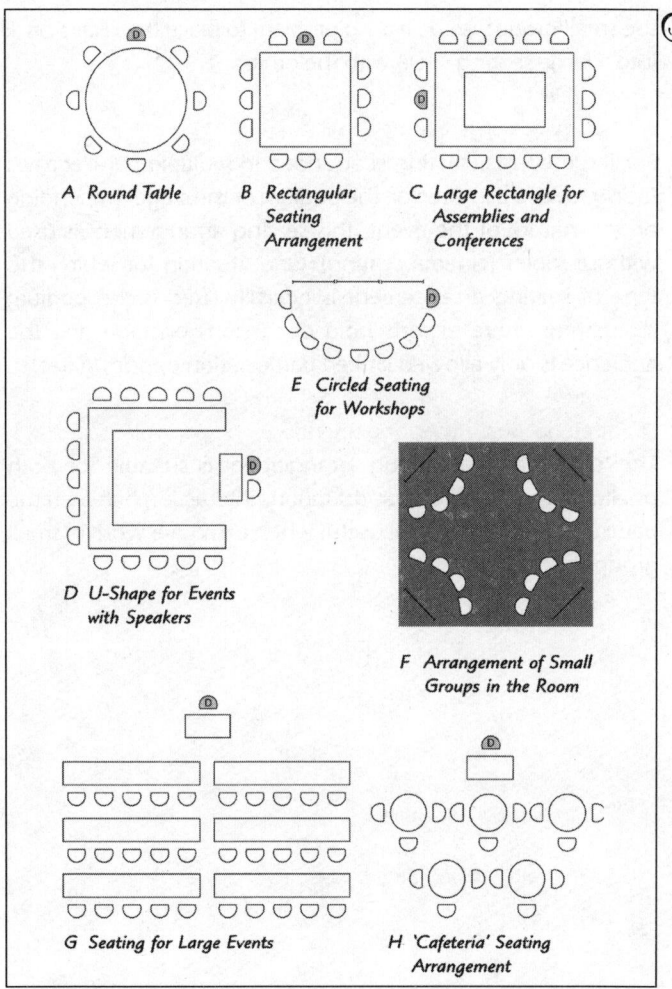

Ill. 5: Various seating arrangements; the letter "D" signifies the position of the meeting director

the small group's work, it is no problem to place the chairs back into a large seating circle with the others.

G Seating for Large Events
For large events, seating is arranged in multiple parallel rows facing toward the director, the podium or the stage. Depending on the nature of the event, this seating arrangement is used without tables (cinema seating). One situation for which this type of seating arrangement is typically used is the podium discussion where experts hold discussions onstage and the audience is only allowed limited participation opportunities.

H "Cafeteria" Seating Arrangement
The 'cafeteria-type' seating arrangement is suitable for both smaller and larger events and supports interaction between the participants. It is above all useful when extensive work in small groups is foreseen.

Part B Execution

As the Meeting Director, you have a decisive influence on the success of the meeting. The essential elements of directing a meeting in professional life – also at the international level – are broadly established and subsequently extensively ritualised. In some types of gatherings, fundamental aspects of direction are also formally established in the form of regulations.

1 Direction of the Course of the Meeting

Your legitimation as the director consists of assuring the proper progression of the meeting. This means that you provide the group with the necessary orientation in the individual stages of the meeting. Ill. 6 depicts the elementary stages of the meeting process.

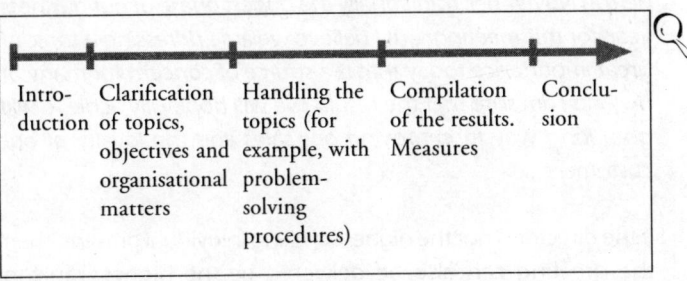

Ill. 6: Stages in the course of a meeting

1.1 The Introduction

In the introductory phase, one should remember that prior to entering the conference room, the participants have usually been preoccupied with something other than the topics of the meeting. Your job as the director at the start is to support the participants and to harmonise the topical matters of the meeting with the other persons present to the greatest extent possible.

By beginning the discussion too directly, the director risks giving the participants the feeling of being overwhelmed, resulting in a subconscious reluctance on their part right at the start. This often manifests itself later in a generally strained atmosphere or in overly critical argument positions.

Primary means of helping to ease the participants' arrival are a friendly, appreciative greeting by the director, a positive acclimatisation into the conference topics, and when advisable, introducing the participants.

An endearing greeting might sound something like this, for instance: *"I would like to cordially welcome you to the first meeting on our project for reducing the complaints rate for our product. Many thanks first off to all of you for taking the time here in November, traditionally the busiest phase of our business year, for this meeting. But I believe we are addressing a topic of great importance today that is a source of concern for many of us. And I am sure that the results we will hopefully achieve will go a long way to improving our sales and the loyalty of our customers. ..."*

If the director is not the highest-ranking individual present, then the greeting can also be delivered by the highest-ranking management figure attending the meeting. This shows the participants which important personality is behind the meeting. The productivity of the meeting will be increased significantly if the host manager states the results that are anticipated right at the start.

Direction of the Course of the Meeting

Here is an overview of the important duties and responsibilities of the Meeting Director in the introductory phase:

Arrangement of the introduction phase

- *Greeting of the participants*
- *Positive general familiarisation with the subject matter*
  Referring to the topical focus gives you the legitimation as the director to redirect the discussion back to the topic at hand in the event of deviations. Nevertheless, do not go into too much detail!
- *Introduction of the participants*
  - *... in the event that they do not know one another*
  - *... in the event that the size of the group allows the time to do so*
  - *The participants can also introduce themselves.*
  - *Especially in the case of new participants, introduction is very important for ensuring that they are readily accepted into the group.*
- *In exceptional situations, however, the introduction should be kept as brief as possible. Examples:*
  - *Announcement of important, unpleasant news*
  - *The discussion of already existing deep conflicts*
  - *In such cases, it is appropriate to move as quickly as possible to establishing the topics for discussion, objectives and to the clarification of organisational matters.*

1.2 Clarification of Topics, Objectives and Organisational Matters

The key points of the meeting are established in this discussion phase. The agenda, which all of the participants should have, is the best basis in this case for mutual planning. It also makes sense to make the agenda generally visible for all the participants on a flip chart, for example. In this way, changes to the order of the topics can be documented in a way that is clear for everyone.

Establishing the topics and objectives is the most important task in this phase. If there is no agenda on hand, then the meeting topics and objectives should be mutually agreed upon this point, and not later. Simply compiling the topics onto a flip chart is usually sufficient in this case.

In addition, this phase should be used to clarify organisational matters, such as the available timeframes. Even if these aspects are already noted in the agenda, surprises still seem to have a habit of popping up on this point: Often, a participant has to leave early for important reasons. This should be known right from the start so that everyone can adjust to the fact that the person in question will not be available from a certain point in time.

> *With an attentive introduction, you make an important contribution to creating a positive discussion climate for the meeting.*

And you will easily recover the time invested in good pre-structuring through the transparency you attain in the procedure and the detours it helps you avoid.

Arrangement of the clarification phase for determination of the topics, objectives and organisational frameworks

- *Clarification of the agenda*
    - *Get confirmation that the agenda sent to everyone contains all the important points*
    - *If need be, discuss and agree on changes of topic*
    - *Clarify the aims of the individual agenda items*

- *If necessary, clarification of the roles in the meeting*
  - Who is the moderator? (If the moderator is not simultaneously the manager present)
  - Who is responsible for the individual topics?
  - Are speakers or experts invited to comment on specific topics?
  - Who is taking the minutes?
- *Clarification of organisational matters*
  - Clarification of the time for ending the meeting (important because of possible subsequent appointments the participants might have, i.e. catching scheduled planes or trains)
  - Break times; if necessary clarify mealtimes
- *Clarification of methods*
  If methods are to be used with which the group is unfamiliar, then a few words should be said on the procedure; however, to avoid an energy-draining discussion on the methods, do not present the work steps in detail.
- *Clarification of any remaining questions the participants might have on the framework of the event*

1.3 Working on the Topics

This phase is at the heart of the meeting. This is where the objectives, problems, opportunities and risks are specified. Now solutions must be sought and various alternatives assessed. Now decisions will be made. Now the discussion will heat up perhaps, requiring you to decisively influence the group as the Meeting Director; or perhaps the exchange of ideas is a little "lukewarm", requiring you to activate the participants.

Important aspects that are decisive in working on the topics consist of ...

- the moderation of participant contributions, direction of the discussion (Part B, Chapter 2)
- the structured procedure in working on the subject matter and problem-solving (Part B, Chapter 3)
- the application of supporting methods, e.g. problem analysis, brainstorming, group work (Part B, Chapter 4.3)
- direction of the group dynamics (Part B, Chapter 6.1)
- dealing with difficult situations and particularities of the participants (Part B, Chapters 7, 8)

Here are some general tips for arranging work on meeting topics:

General tips for working on subject matter

- *To familiarise the participants with a topic,* **it is recommended to get everyone's standard of knowledge "on the same page".** *An expert could initially give a brief content overview on the topic.*
- *The* **agenda items** *should be* clearly delineated from one another. *A compilation of the results at the end of the discussion on a particular topic can provide a clean conclusion.*
- *One should fundamentally* stay with an agenda item until a result has been reached that can realistically be achieved. *If important ancillary aspects of a topic arise during the discussion that are nevertheless not central to the meeting at hand or if new meeting points are recommended, then you should collect these in a "topic repository", for example on the flip chart. The participants now know that the new point will not be forgotten.*
- Measures and individual results *that have been agreed on by the group of participants should be* documented immediately.
- *In* meetings occurring on a cyclical basis, **work on the topic(s) should begin with the reading of the minutes from the last meeting:** *The*

participants inform one another regarding the extent to which the measures discussed in the previous meeting have been implemented.

1.4 Compilation of Results – Measures

All agenda items have been dealt with. The group has agreed on results. Activities and tasks have additionally been agreed upon and documented on the flip chart. Everyone feels like everything that is functionally possible has been accomplished in this meeting. Now it is time for the group director to lead the group back out of the work. Above all, this means reviewing what has been accomplished for the group and ensuring that the agreed-upon results can move into implementation.

It can make sense, particularly after longer meetings, to have another look at the measures plan with all of the agreed-upon measures. This serves three primary functions:

- Some of the topics addressed can be linked with one another; during the course of the discussion, it can sometimes occur that measures agreed to later on place in question other measures agreed to earlier. Often affiliated activities can be bundled and taken care of by the same responsible party.
- Some meetings see so many measures agreed upon that it is doubtful whether they can all be realised. It is not the job of the director to question the agreed-upon results, but he or she should ask whether activity planning is realistic ("Hygiene Check").
- An overview of the agreed measures clarifies the actual value of what has been accomplished for the participants; this can alleviate the feeling of regret for having spent so much time in the meeting.

> **Result compilation and measures planning – important aspects that should be clarified now**
>
> - *What are the most important results and decisions **that the group has come up with?***
> - *Are the agreed-upon measures …*
>   - *– capable of being realised,*
>   - *– acceptable **(even at second glance)**,*
>   - *– coordinated?*
> - *Is anything missing?*
> - *When and how will the participants receive the minutes of the meeting?*
> - *Who has to be informed about the results other than the participants?*
> - *When should the group meet again?*

1.5 The Conclusion

The participants should leave the conference in the best possible mood. The emotional aftertaste of a meeting often stays around longer than the actual results achieved. Of course, things do not always go well. As the director, you should give a summary that acknowledges what has occurred in the most appreciative and simultaneously honest way – whatever has occurred.

If the meeting runs positively, then for example you can refer to …
- the good preparation of the gathering
- the abundance and quality of the results achieved
- the care given to the problem analysis
- the wealth of ideas from the participants

Direction of the Course of the Meeting

- the willingness to compromise on the part of the participants
- the appreciative nature of the dealings with one another
- the interesting, lively brief presentations made, and much more

But you can also acknowledge a meeting that is proven to be of a more critical nature in a sensible manner. You can refer to …
- the very open, courageous statements
- the controversial, interesting discussion
- the advantage, ultimately taken, of the opportunity to openly articulate resentments
- the emergence of fundamental obstacles in problem-solving that can be worked on, now that they have been recognised
- the justified question as to whether the group will be able to actually manage the tasks at hand if it continues to work in the previous fashion

Your summary should not be perceived to be pretending things are better than they actually are and it should not offend anyone personally. Without prejudice, you should allow yourself to feel the palpable atmosphere in the room and then name it in a constructive manner. Teams that value good communication and that continually seek to improve their conference practise often close their meetings with a short debriefing analysis:
- In a "closing flashlight", the participants briefly state one after another what they liked and where they see room for improvement next time (Part B, Chapter 2.8).
- Using a "closing flip", this assessment can also be visualised: Each of the participants sticks an adhesive dot onto a "Satisfaction Scale"; in conclusion, they each comment on their assessment (Part B, Chapter 4.2).

Arrangement of a conclusion to a meeting

- *Compilation* of the results and the process by the director
- *Expression of thanks* to the participants for their contributions
- Perhaps a *"closing flashlight"*: the director's summarising process appraisal should come at the end
- Bidding *farewell* to the participants; the last word should be left to the director who is to make the closing summary of the results

2 Meeting Direction as a Moderation Task

Constructive meeting direction begins and ends with the moderator supporting and simplifying the communication within the group. You can easily tell by the reactions of the participants whether they find your directive function helpful in this regard.

The most important thing for this is that the director has a clear "internal image" of the course of the meeting as described above in the individual phases. If this progression is clear to the director, then he or she can guide the group through the meeting in a relaxed fashion, always providing the catalyst when the communication flow encounters obstacles.

The following compilation contains a series of important intervention forms for moderators. These represent the elementary tools of the Meeting Director.

2.1 Giving the Floor

Give the floor in the order of the requests to speak. – This may be the most fundamental direction activity in group discussions. Even the quieter participants know that they will be heard when they raise their hand to speak. An atmosphere of fairness and relaxation is the result.

If several participants signal their requests in rapid succession, try to remember the order. With a larger number of requests, you can note the order on paper (list of speakers).

In giving the floor to participants, use a standard formulation like: *"Ms Miller, please."* By refraining from comments or valuating undertones in giving the floor, you demonstrate your neutrality.

"Queue-jumpers" who simply begin speaking whether it is their turn or not are easily blocked: *"I believe Ms Miller was before you."*

The participants begin to depend on your direction of the meeting. The aggression level in the group sinks.

Register the speaking requests of the group members precisely (eye contact!) and validate them. High-ranking participants who are present are usually appreciative of a fair form of granting the floor. They wait their turn and then take the time and space that they need to appropriately state their position. However, if such persons unexpectedly fail to observe the speaking order, then your experience must guide you on a case-by-case basis in deciding whether to permit the higher-ranking participants to have the right-of-way or to respectfully intervene.

Under certain circumstances, allow direct objections.

There is no rule without an exception! There are times when you should deviate from the order of the speaking requests; namely, when a participant addresses his or her comment directly to another participant, for example, by criticising the other. In this case, the person who the comment is addressed to should receive the opportunity to respond directly to what has been said. As the director, you can insert the objection in this way: *"Mr Meier's comments were addressed directly to you, Mr Schulz. I presume that you would like to respond?"*

If, for his part, Mr Schulz now addresses Mr Meier personally, for instance, to deliver a justification or a counterattack, then you can also permit him to make a statement outside the boundaries of the list of speakers. However, afterwards you should redirect the discussion back into the group to avoid having the objections take over the subject matter: *"I have the impression that the two of you could provide one another with some important information. With your permission, it is now Ms Bauer's turn. She made her request some time ago."*

Meeting Direction as a Moderation Task

If the topics discussed in the objections are important for all of the participants, then you can include the entire group in the discussion: *"How does the problem discussed by Mr Schulz and Mr Meier affect the other working areas?"* Afterwards you return to the original topic or to the order contained in the list of speakers.

2.2 Posing Questions

Support the process with questions. – It is the job of the director to organise the discussion process and to create space for solutions, but not to take personal responsibility for the solution to the existing problem. It usually leads quickly to the isolation of the moderator if this person also assumes the role of the expert who wants to tell the group what it should do. Admittedly, the exception to this is when the moderator is simultaneously a manager representing certain positions in the meeting.

By using questions, you, as the moderator, can open doors and promote problem-solving.

Benefits of questions in meetings

- *Questions increase the information base for problem-solving*
- *They open doors for creative viewpoints and new ideas*
- *They activate the meeting participants*
- *They help to structure the work on the topics*
- *They help to make it possible to talk about the feelings and needs of the participants*
- *They help to dissolve blockades*

Depending on the situation, experienced moderators use very different questioning methods and go with the energies of the group in this way, instead of attempting to use questioning techniques to prescribe a solution method. Here are some helpful questioning methods for conducting meetings:

Questions Regarding Facts:
- "What market share does competitor X have in this sector?"
- *"How high are the costs that we have to save in the upcoming year?"*

Questions Regarding Context and Effects:
- "When does the problem not occur?"
- "What other work sectors does the success of our project depend on?"

Questions Regarding Explanations, Estimates and Perceptions:
- "What do you see as the explanation for both construction departments working in such an uncoordinated way?"
- "What is your perception of the current mood of the customers?"

Questions Regarding Forecasts:
- "How do you think the customer structure will change in the next few years?"
- "What topics will be important for our team in one or two years?"

Questions Regarding Objectives:
- "What requirements should the new software meet?"
- "What sales do we want to generate with the new product line in the upcoming year?"

Questions Regarding Solutions:
- "What has already been tried to solve the problem? How successful was it?"
- "What can you imagine as an alternative concept?"

Commitment Questions, Questions Regarding Responsibilities:
- "Can I record this now as the result of our discussion?"
- *"Which one of you would be willing to get the necessary offers from the suppliers?"*

Three Special Types of Questions

Scale Questions

With scale questions, one sets numeric values – e.g. a scale from 0 to 10 – in relation to certain circumstances, problems, feelings or expectations. This makes situations more firmly comprehensible and tangible in their dynamics.

Examples:
- "On a scale of 1 to 100, how satisfied are we at the moment with the situation in the Sales Department?"
- "On a scale of ... to ..., how close have we come to finding a good solution for the problem?"

On the basis of scale questions, you can also clearly express the value of small improvements, as well as introducing slight catalysts for change – something like this: *"What do we have to do to increase our satisfaction with the Sales Department by five points on our scale?"*

The scale evaluation can be conducted verbally or you can have the participants visualise them with adhesive dots on the flip chart (cp. Part B, Chapter 4.2).

Questions Regarding Specifics / Inquiring Questions

Questions on specifics and inquiring questions help to make situations comprehensible for everyone present. With their help, unspoken assumptions can be laid open, and they are additionally a good means to break through blockades in the process:

Participant statement:	*"We'll never be able to do it like that."*
Specification question in response:	*"What do you mean with 'like that'?"*
Participant statement:	*"Our customers will never accept that."*
Inquiring question:	*"What makes you so sure that our customers won't go along?"*

The "Miracle Question"

The "miracle question" was made famous by psychotherapist and scientist Steve de Shazer. He established that clients – just like organisations – often express their desires for a change in any given situation in very unspecific terms. They hope for *"better communication"* or *"less friction with one another"* or *"more satisfaction"*. The "miracle question" helps to be more precise about hopes and expectations: *"Imagine that one night while you are asleep a miracle happens and your problem was solved. How would you notice? How would your colleagues find out without you saying a word about it to them?"*

At this point, the participants usually now begin to develop internal images of the desired circumstances. Ask the participants to describe these images. The layout of the desired situation can then be used for the specific formulation of the working objective.

There are also unproductive question forms that you would be better off avoiding:

> **Inappropriate question forms – avoid ...**

- *Suggestive questions:* **"Don't you also want to avoid an unnecessary expansion of the project?"**
- *Teacher questions / Knowledge questions:* **"So, which of you has really internalised the new 'Business Terms and Conditions'?"**

- *Questions that lead someone to lose face:* "*So, is there anyone here who hasn't gone through the minutes of the last meeting yet?*"
- *Justification questions:* "*Why didn't you get around to it earlier?*"
- *Killer questions:* "*Which of you don't care anyway how the new break room is designed?*"

2.3 Active Listening

Concentrated listening is one of the most effective and at the same time one of the most subtle tools of moderation. While participants are expressing their thoughts, reacting to one another, etc., you should be able to restrain yourself. Let the effect of what is said come through and note the emotions and energies that are at work in the group. Take notice of how the meeting participants see things. You receive a clear impression of the facts and sensibilities and you can also experience the relationship dynamics between the individual participants. This allows you to pose the right questions to keep things moving and to cushion imbalances in the interactions.

Perhaps you notice the tendency of one participant to subtly detract a quieter participant. To balance this, you can inconspicuously encourage the reserved participant to articulate their position more clearly, long before it comes to a conflict or frustration.

The tools of active listening

- *Scheduling enough time to also bear with moments of silence*
- *Concentrating fully on the group*
- *Ensuring that you keep the entire group in view*
- *Using inquiring questions and encouragement to prompt participants to delve more deeply into particular aspects:* "*I think that's very interesting*

for everyone; could you tell us in more detail about your experiences with supplier X."

- *Being impartial; making no judgements*
- *Allowing participants to speak until they are finished*

2.4 Reformulating Statements, Introducing Compilations

The ability to briefly recap statements made by participants in a meeting is one of the most important skills that you should use as a Meeting Director.

When you repeat in your own words the information and estimates articulated by a participant, you can ...

- ensure that you have understood the viewpoint of the participant correctly and prevent misunderstandings
- show your respect to the participant
- work out important aspects for further discussion
- relieve conflict situations by slowing things down (cp. Part B, Chapter 2.6)

Important aspects of repeating participant statements

- *Arranging the repetition of what was said appropriately – from condensing it into one word up to recapping complex thought processes.*
- *Repeating to give the participant the opportunity to correct you – Example: "If I've understood you correctly, ..."*
- *Avoiding (negative) valuations and irony, such as, "You don't seriously think that the ..."*
- *Your repetition is successful if the participant in question signals their approval.*

Sometimes meetings can lose their intended point. If this happens, the moderator should introduce compilations from a longer portion of the meeting: *"In short, what positions have been represented (for example, pro and con) in the last ten minutes?"*

Compilations ...
- show where the group is
- can direct the attention to important matters that have not yet been considered
- often serve as guideposts for the further course of the meeting

Example: *"Up to now, we've only looked at the opportunities and acceptable costs of a new product line. We haven't yet discussed whether we have enough personnel resources for the construction and the tests."*

2.5 Offer a Change of Focus

When central topics have been overseen in the course of discussion up to now, you can change the focus of the discussion. You can introduce new questions. For this, you need the consent of the group, of course. And to get it, you can use the following three-step technique:

Three steps to changing the focus

1. *A description of what the group is doing at the moment*
   (Introduce a compilation, reformulate statements – see above)
2. *Give a recommendation for a new direction of the discussion*
   "Up until now, we haven't given question XY any consideration at all; maybe we should have a closer look at this aspect."
3. *Obtain the consent of the group*
   "Is that agreeable to everybody?"
   "Does this sound like a sensible way to proceed?"

If the group agrees, then you can direct the discussion on the new viewpoint. If not, you can use the same method again to clarify how to proceed with the group:

1. Description: *"I see that viewpoint XY is not such a central issue for you at the moment."*
2. Recommendation: *"I suggest that we first compile the points that you still want to clarify today so that we can continue to progress on our project."*
3. Obtaining Consent: *"Is that agreeable?"*

2.6 Reframing

Reframing means reformulating negative formulations describing problem situations in a constructive way, giving them a new, solution-oriented "frame".

Positive rephrasing can elegantly cushion harsh comments, particularly when participants are "on a rant".

Example

Participant statement: *"The employees in Orders Received are just plain lazy; often enough you can't get anyone on the phone, even if you let it ring ten times."*

Reframing: *"I think you've made an important point in bringing up the importance of the telephone presence. In your opinion, our colleagues have a relaxed attitude regarding the phones. What can we do so that they recognise how important it is to react right away to calls?"*

Of course, one should not overdo reframing. It is easy to lose credibility when one suddenly begins diplomatically reinterpreting every "problem" as a "challenge" or "opportunity". What is important is to stay in tune with the group and in contact with its perception of reality.

2.7 Tactful Blocking

In almost every meeting, we meet personalities whose speaking contributions seem to never want to end, while other participants are sneaking glances at their watches probably thinking, *"Actually the moderator should be intervening here"*. What to do?

- First Possibility: Allow it
  - Opportunity: After having made a few "speeches", the participant in question has run out of things to say and will accordingly begin to participate in a less verbal fashion.
  - Risk: Since no one is objecting, the "speechmaker" feels encouraged to continue with the elaborate approach.
- Second Possibility: Blocking
  - Opportunity: The group can soon begin again to work on its topics in a disciplined manner.
  - Risk: The "speechmaker" feels devalued and begins to explain his or her conduct or, worse, seeks a conflict with the moderator. This is then a genuine obstacle to proceeding with the actual work.

Based on experience, it usually backfires if the moderator fails to counter an inappropriately longwinded individual. Generally speaking, the group ostensibly appears to accept the laissez faire style of the moderator, but the subsequent meeting feedback round usually packs a surprise punch. The moderator is now reprimanded for failing to exert more control over the process. Therefore the following recommendation:

> *If individual participants demand too much speaking time to the detriment of the meeting's progress, you should intervene. But by no means should you embarrass the overly enthusiastic speaker.*

Call for a break during the course of the person's address or carefully merge into his or her flow of speech. It is of utmost importance that your first words to the interrupted participant make it plain that you appreciate him or her personally and that you take their contribution seriously. Say something like ...

- the participant has just touched on an important point, namely XY, and that it makes sense to reflect on this point with the entire group – then ask the group for their comments.
- the participant has just introduced a wealth of interesting viewpoints. Ask him or her if it is OK to work on these now together. Then refer to one of the aspects that were addressed and open up the discussion to the group again.
- you want to record the points mentioned so that they are not lost in the continued discussion. Write these points down from memory on the flip chart and ask the participant whether you have correctly repeated the central aspects. Then continue with the moderation and bring the group back into the discussion.

Both the group and the "speechmaker" will register that you are actively directing the meeting without having to become impolite. This increases the trust in your competence as a director.

2.8 Flashlight Rounds

After longer meeting phases or at the end of the meeting, it is recommended to conduct a mutual assessment. Since the degree of involvement of each of the individual participants in the discussion is usually varied, it is important to repeatedly create space where all of the participants are of equal importance. The moderator's request for the participants to comment one after the other on a particular question or on their current feelings helps to stabilise the balance of forces and to bring important aspects to the surface that have previously been suppressed.

A flashlight round generally runs as follows:
1. The moderator asks the group to comment on a specific question. Depending on the focus, this could include questions such as:
   - *"How would you assess our current progress on the project?"*
   - *"How are you feeling at the moment about our discussion?"*
2. The participants now comment one after another (for example, in the order of the seating arrangement) on the subject matter.

Principles for conducting a flashlight round are:
- The comments should be kept brief.
- The comments should not be discussed or commented on further; only questions to ensure proper understanding of the statement are permissible.

In many cases, a flashlight round can stand on its own. Often however, it can be taken as an occasion to address dynamics that have not yet received adequate attention or to add new topics to the agenda.

3 Provide Structure

Particularly in the initial phase, the group of participants often needs orientation – not just in regard to the organisational framework, but also in relation to the manner in which the topics at issue can be worked on. More than anything else, the objectives listed in the agenda for each agenda item (Part A, Chapter 3.2) clarify what is expected of the participants in the discussion (for example, ideas) and what is not expected (for example, decisions).

One essential job of the moderator consists of establishing the current extent to which a topic is actually being handled, e.g. whether the problem has already been precisely registered and whether ideas for its solution have already been presented.

3.1 Problem-Solving Procedure

One practicable possibility for providing the group with structure is the orientation of the problem-solving phases.

Five steps of problem-solving

1. *Analysing the problem and previous solution attempts*
   - *"What is the nature of the problem?"*
   - *"How is the problem demonstrated today and what is the desired objective?" (Target-Actual Analysis)*
2. *Collecting solution alternatives – brainstorming*
   - *"What solution options are available?"*
   - *"Are there alternatives that we have not considered yet?"*
3. *Evaluating alternatives*
   - *"What criteria should we apply to the decision?"*
   - *"How do we prioritise these criteria?"*

4. *Decision meeting*
    - *"Can we agree to a mutual procedure?"*
    - *"Can we adhere to initially trying solution plan X?"*
5. *Agreeing on specific measures*
    - *"What specific first steps should we agree on?"*
    - *"Who is assuming the responsibility for which activities?"*

As the moderator, you can recommend the following guidelines to the group:
- Only start looking for solutions when everyone has agreed on what the problem is.
- Keep the brainstorming phase clearly separated from the evaluation phase – appraisals of ideas, corrections and criticism that come too early undermine the willingness of the participants to involve themselves creatively.
- During the course of the meeting, direct the energies toward solutions. Accusations and excuses lead to nothing but a deterioration of the discussion atmosphere.

Display confidence as the moderator that, basically, there is a solution and that the only question is a matter of what the solution is, but be reserved with your own solution ideas.

This reinforces the consciousness of the meeting participants to be responsible for finding the solution themselves. If you still want to introduce new aspects, you can formulate your ideas as questions (*"Have you thought about...?"*, *"Could X also be an alternative?"*). This maintains the group's role as the "author" of its own story.

3.2 Work Phases in Workshop Moderation

In some clarification processes, the actual problem is still "unfocused" and not precisely defined. The jury, so to speak, is still out regarding what is important and what can be put "on the back burner" at the moment. Such situations generally tend to represent a workshop rather than a classic meeting. In such cases, a precise agenda often emerges within the framework of the event itself. The structure of such workshops should therefore be designed in an open manner, so that the participants can define relevant subject matter without pressure and agree on a manner of procedure. An orientation on eight work phases has proved to be a reliable way of proceeding:

Eight workshop work phases

1. *Introduction*
   - *Communication of the objective/assignment framework of the event*
   - *Organisational matters*
   - *Participant introduction if appropriate*
   - *Clarification of the roles and the method*
2. *Producing problem-orientation*
   - *Registering the sensibilities of the participants in relation to the problem (e.g. "How important is the topic for our daily work?")*
3. *Compiling topics*
   - *Creating a topic/problem repository*
   - *Compiling sub-topics into topic complexes*
4. *Prioritising topics*
   - *Defining the relevant priority criteria (for example, urgency, responsibility, degree of applicability to the participants)*
   - *Prioritising*
   - *Agreeing on specific subject matter for the next work phase*
5. *Finding solutions*

Provide Structure

- *Clarifying the working setting (e.g. plenum or small group)*
- *Clarification and realisation of logical partial work steps*
- *In group work: Presentation of the group results in the plenum with a closing discussion*

6. *Evaluating and deciding on solutions*
   - *Choosing an evaluation procedure – for instance, majority vote or applying a decision matrix*
   - *Making a decision*

7. *Agreement of measures – safeguarding results*
   - *Creating a measures plan*
   - *Agreements for reviewing the success of the meeting*

8. *Closing*
   - *Documenting questions that remain open*
   - *Collecting feedback on the workshop*

You will find many suggestions for the practical form of the eight work phases sketched out here in Part B, Chapter 4.2.

4 Moderation Techniques and Visualisations in Support of the Process

Many people find it much easier to assimilate information when it is optically visible. One speaks in this regard of visual learning types. Therefore, a significant recent innovation in our meeting culture is the invention of the moderation method developed in the 1970's: visual discussion using key-word scripted cards attached to pinboards. The issue in moderation is getting the right balance between verbal dialogue and visual support, so that we also maintain eye contact with one another instead of simply gazing spellbound at flip charts and pinboards.

Let's take a look first at the media that can be used for visualisation.

4.1 Media in Group Communication

We will start with a genuine classic in meeting media, universally applicable, mobile and on hand in virtually every meeting room, the ...

Flip Chart

The flip chart can be used flexibly, since it only requires a couple of thick felt tip markers for writing or drawing. Use of the flip chart generally thrives on the spontaneous activity of the Meeting Director or a participant making a presentation.

Possibilities for Usage:
- Presenting prepared texts and visualisations (for example, agenda, graphics)
- Documenting questions, results and agreements during the meeting

Moderation Techniques and Visualisations

- Maintaining what has been worked out in a visible form (the sheets can be affixed to the walls with masking tape)
- Noting newly emerging topics on the flip chart so that they can be worked on later

Please observe:
- How well the medium is received depends significantly on the quality of the handwriting
- Corrections in the text and graphics leave traces or are quite troublesome

Transforming one's normal handwriting into suitable flip chart handwriting is an important matter for Meeting Directors, often requiring a compromise to be found between attractive handwriting and quick handwriting.

Here are the most important basics for appropriate writing on a flip chart:
- Use upper and lower case, font size approximately 1 to 1 1/5 inches
- Squeeze your letters close together (makes a more attractive optical impression and saves space)
- Leave one to two finger-widths of space between lines
- Whenever possible, do not use more than two font sizes or more than two colours (clarity)

Tips for using a flip chart

- *Each sheet needs a heading*
- *Record as few units of information on one sheet as possible*
- *Err on the side of writing too big rather than too small*
- *Do not speak when writing, as you should always face the audience when speaking*

Pinboard and Moderation Materials

The pinboard or moderation board can be used above all in workshops. Its core element is usually a large foam rubber panel attached to a free-standing metal frame, making it mobile. Before using them, pinboards should be fitted with large sheets of packaging paper. Provisionally attached moderation cards can be permanently stuck to the packaging paper sheets later with a glue stick so that the sheets, including the cards, can simply be rolled up and transported.

Possibilities for Usage:
- Conducting "card surveys" with the group (see Part B, Chapter 4.2)
- Visualising complex correlations in a step-by-step fashion
- Presenting fully prepared depictions of complex matters
- A documentation medium for group work
- A room partition when several small groups are working in one room
- An attachment surface for transparencies, flip chart sheets, drawings, wall news sheets

Please observe:

The conditions for working with pinboards are similar to working with a flip chart: Since the medium is used mostly for handwritten text and sketches, the result is generally vivid, but not optically perfect.

Along with pinboards, you should also keep the following materials on hand if you want to moderate meeting sequences:
- Moderation cards in various shapes and sizes
- Felt tip markers in various colours and thicknesses
- Adhesive dots (for the group to use in prioritising and assessing topics)

- Pins
- Pin cushions
- Glue sticks
- Masking tape (for affixing packaging paper sheets to the wall)
- Scissors

Handwriting for moderation cards is subject to the same recommendations as for writing on a flip chart, but the font size should be somewhat smaller. A moderation card should not contain more than three lines of text.

Overhead Projectors and Beamers

Overhead projectors and beamers are the most popular media for conveying trends, key data and concepts. The picture is focused and bright, and with beamers in particular, which are broadly accepted as a presentation standard, you can simplify the registration of information by using animations.

Possibilities for Usage:
- Conveying fully prepared information (in text, graphics)
- Documenting meeting results in real-time (writing on blank transparencies or creating simultaneous minutes on a laptop)

Please observe:
- The brightness of the projection surface occupies a portion of the attention, with the picture becoming the focus; the people watching easily lose sight of one another.
- Fan noises can be disruptive and tiring for the participants.
- As a rule, the participants can scarcely be actively involved and therefore fall to some degree into "consumer role" (in contrast to the flip chart, where you actually go "centre-stage" to write or draw something).

Presenting in front of an international team

> *How would you go about giving a presentation at a meeting with international business partners?*

The first step is to be aware of your own style and the effect it might have on other people. It is difficult and probably not desirable to try to imitate another style but you can try to limit or build on elements of your own style according to how you think the audience might react. A German presenter might, for instance, leave out some historical background and detail when presenting to a US audience.

In any situation it can also help to show the audience that you are aware of your cultural background and that they may have a different style.

It is important to adapt your language to your team. If you are speaking in English, make sure that it is understandable for your audience.

Here are some tips on how to do this:
- Avoid idioms, i.e. phrases that have a figurative meaning and cannot be understood literally
- Speak more slowly and clearly than you might do with native speakers
- Stress important words
- Make your structure clear to the audience
- Check whether the audience is following your arguments
- Support your argument with visuals

It pays to continuously work on professionalizing one's own presentation skills: Phases of mutual information exchange in meetings can be arranged in a more interesting fashion; well-prepared information allows you to work on more complexity in the meeting, and you will profit in the result of better problem-solving.

Tips for using overhead projectors and beamers

Arranging charts:
- *Create the fewest possible number of charts*
- *It is better to use the diagonal format than the vertical one*
- *Give each chart a heading*
- *Keywords or phrases are better than continuous text*
- *Select a simple font of adequate size*
- *Only use core statements; spread complex content over several transparency sheets*
- *Use pictures and graphic elements*
- *Use colours and animations sparingly*

Presentation tips:
- *When explaining, lead the audience through the chart and maintain contact with the audience; do not talk to the wall*
- *With an overhead projector: Avoid using the overlap technique (also called the "Striptease" technique, meaning covering the content of the transparencies and then "revealing" it during the course of the explanation – the participants feel a little deprived by the initial withholding of information)*
  Alternative: Spread the information over several transparencies
- *With a beamer: Partial aspects should be introduced into a chart gradually*

Tips for the moderator/meeting director:
- *Agree on a time limit prior to the presentation (if possible, no longer than ten minutes; more turns a meeting into a presentation event)*
- *Clarify prior to the presentation whether questions and comments during the presentation are desired or whether the dialogue should first be opened up afterwards (Tip: Allow questions regarding understanding of the information to be answered during the presentation, while comments and discussion are to be left until afterwards)*

4.2 Work and Visualisation Techniques for Groups

The work techniques depicted here represent a methodical repertoire for the effective, interesting arrangement of a meeting. This depiction is oriented on the sequence of the phases in arranging workshops (see Part B, Chapter 3).

Introduction

1. Public Opinion Barometer

Application situations:
- The work climate plays a large role for the group and/or the meeting topic
- The sensibilities and feelings are currently unclear

The group should be fundamentally familiar with visualisations and demonstrate a willingness to articulate feelings right at the start (otherwise there is the risk that they will feel overwhelmed by the procedure or simply reject it).

Procedure:

The participants are invited to stick a dot onto the prepared chart (see below). In the introductory phase, the moderator can ask the participants to use the adhesive dots to comment on their state of mind.

Moderation Techniques and Visualisations

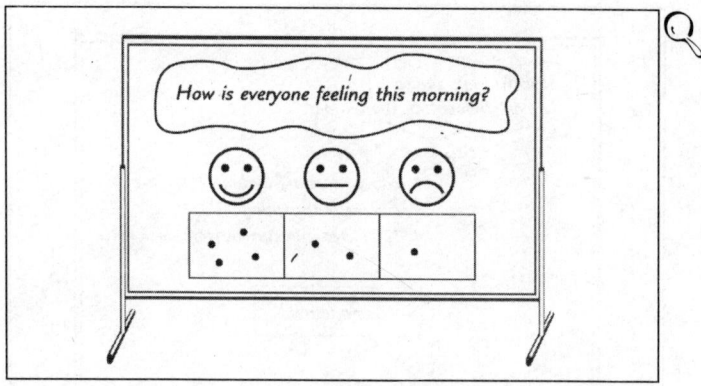

Ill. 7: Public opinion barometer – Example

2. Task Triangle

Application situations:
- The interests of different participants should/must be taken into consideration in the meeting
- The group fears hidden agendas (dictated from "upstairs")

Procedure:
The moderator draws the triangle with the designations of the persons/groups involved in the overall process on the flip chart or on the pinboard. He or she then introduces the predefined points (for example, assignment from Executive Management) to the group. In conclusion, the moderator clarifies and visualises the roles of the remaining players with the participants and comes up with meeting objectives together with the group.

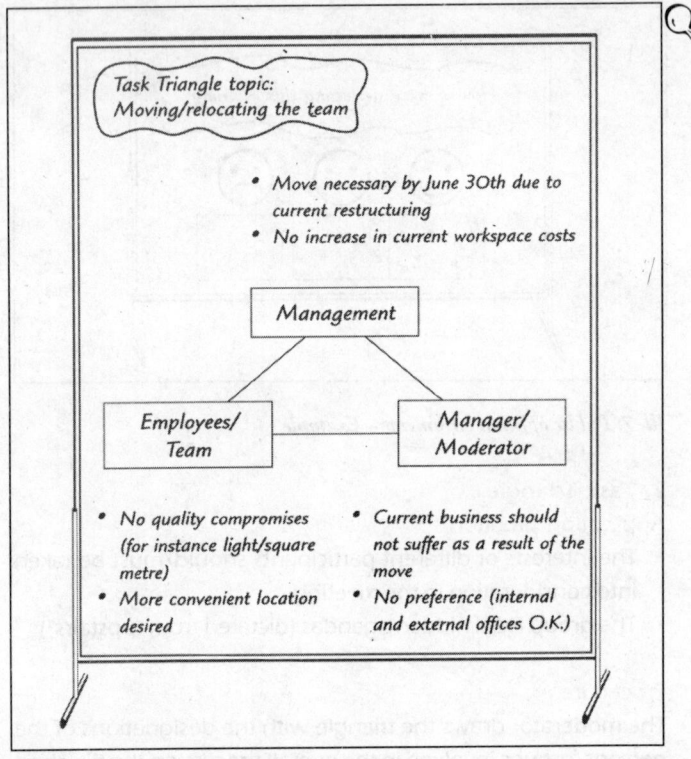

Ill. 8: Example of a task triangle

Creating Problem-Orientation – Visualising Theories and Scale Questions (One-Point Question)

Application situations:
- The problem is ill-defined
- The meaning of the topic is to be explained
- The viewpoints of the participants in regard to the topic are not generally known

Moderation Techniques and Visualisations

Procedure:

The moderator prepares a chart with a thesis or a question and also featuring a scale (see Part B, Chapter 2.2), then explains the thesis or question to the participants and asks them to depict their assessment visually with an adhesive dot. After everyone present has added their dot, the director opens the discussion by asking for comments on the dots. The comments themselves can also be visualised. Work involving visualising theses and scale questions generally creates a very lively, interesting discussion.

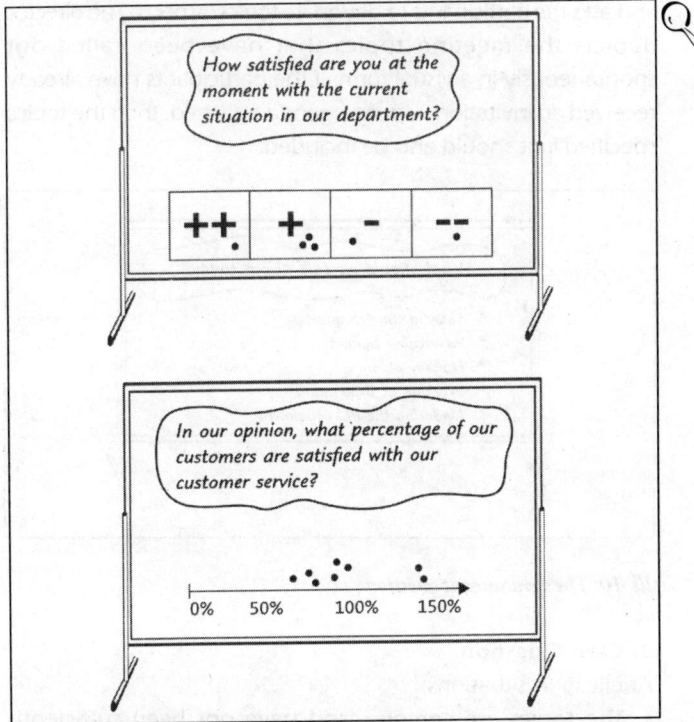

Ill. 9: Examples of visualising theses and scale questions

Compiling Topics

1. Spontaneous Questions

Application situations:

- The agenda items have yet to be established
- Additions to the agenda are to be anticipated
- The agenda has not yet been agreed

Procedure:

The moderator writes a heading or question onto the flip chart and asks the participants to designate topics/aspects. The director depicts the meeting topics that have been called out spontaneously in a visual form. If the participants have already received an invitation with an agenda attached, then the topics specified in it should also be included.

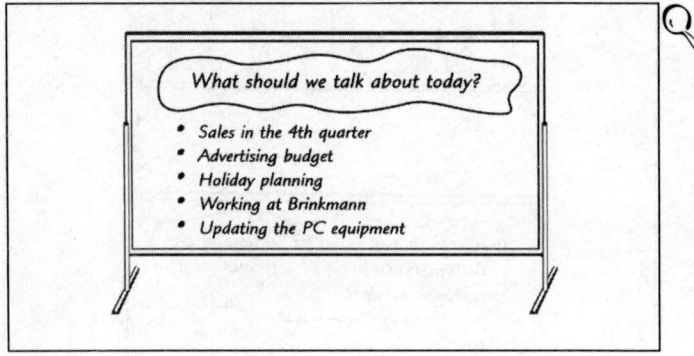

Ill. 10: The spontaneous question

2. Card Question

Application situations:

- The topics are complex and have not been sufficiently structured yet

Moderation Techniques and Visualisations

- The group's full range of opinions should be depicted
- A consideration phase is necessary prior to an answer
- There is enough time available (approximately 30–45 min.)

Procedure:
- The moderator attaches a card with his or her question to an empty pinboard and then explains the question
- Cards and felt tip markers are distributed
- The participants write on the cards:
  - Only write one thought per card
  - Write legibly
  - If the work is conducted with large groups or time is short, it can make sense to provide a guideline for the number of contributions per participant ("... the two to three most important thoughts on ...")
- The moderator collects the cards
- He reads the cards out aloud and shows them to the group
- After each card, the group calls out the aspect of the topic that the card should be allocated to. The sorting criteria should be worked out by the group. If the participants cannot agree, then the author should decide on the allocation of the card.
- Each card is pinned to the moderation board according to its allocation, resulting in card groupings ("clusters") over the surface of the pinboard
- Each cluster receives a heading. The clusters are circled in with a line. The heading is noted on a moderation card and filed with the corresponding cluster.

Now the topics that have emerged can be worked on in order, or the topics can be prioritised first (see next section).

Card questions provide a good introduction to an intensive work phase.

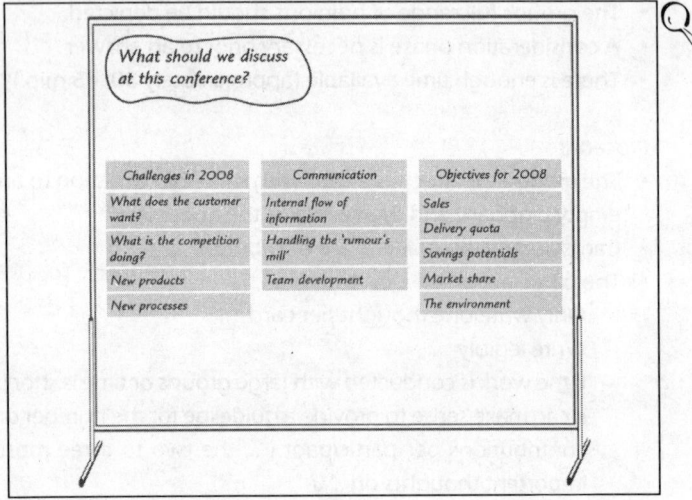

Ill. 11: The card question

Prioritising and Selecting Topics – Multi-faceted Prioritising Question

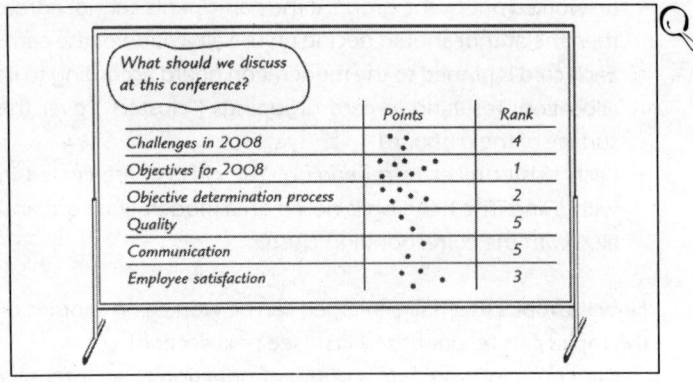

Ill. 12: Examples of prioritising questions

Moderation Techniques and Visualisations

Application situations:
- It is not yet clear for the participants what priority the topics have
- The available time is not sufficient to address all the desired topics with in the conference

Procedure:
The topics and the specific prioritising question are visualised on the flip chart. The moderator explains the question and discusses prioritising criteria with the participants, such as ...

- Importance (*"For which topics do we have a clear assignment for change? What will have the most enduring effect?"*)
- Urgency (*"What has to be done right away?"*)
- Responsibility (*"Which topics are our responsibility?"*)
- Resources (*"For which topics are solutions affordable?"*)
- Participants are personally affected (*"Which topics do we have the greatest amount of solution energy for?"*)
- Know-how (*"Which topics do we have the necessary skills for?"*)

Each of the participants then receives several adhesive dots that can be allocated to the suggested work topics.

Rule of thumb: Divide the number of topics by two (e.g. with six topics, each participant gets three adhesive dots). It is important that all of the participants stick up their dots more or less simultaneously so that individual participants are not able to "strategically" tip the scales in the end.

Finding Solutions

1. Herringbone Diagram (Cause & Effect Diagram)

Application situations:

- There is a problem (mistake, shortcoming, predicament)
- The causes of the problem are not yet known
- The problem is poorly structured

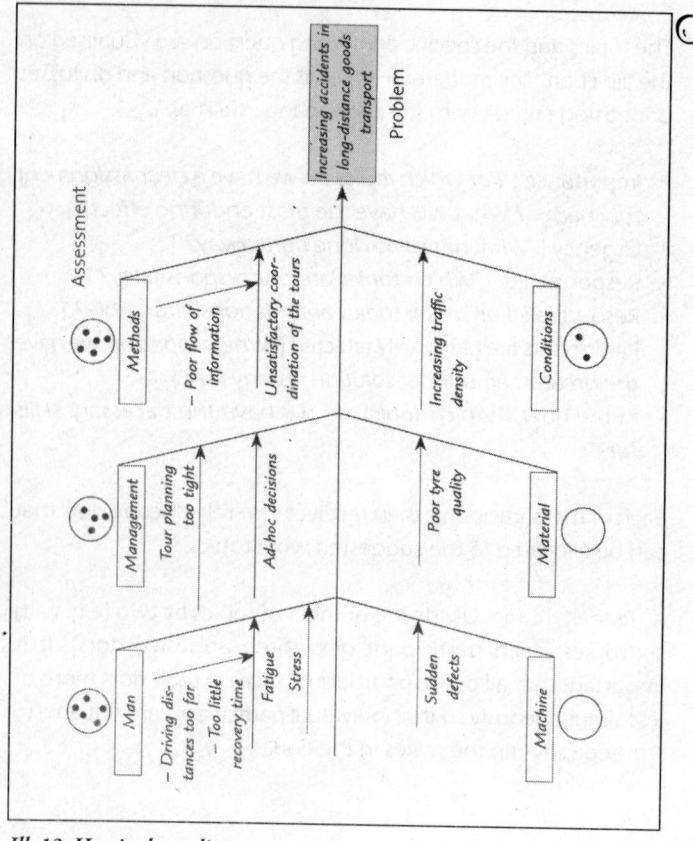

Ill. 13: Herringbone diagram

Procedure:
The moderator creates a visual of the analysis scheme framework which resembles a herringbone pattern. Then questions are posed exploring the causes of a problem in six different areas (6 M), namely ...

- Man (knowledge, experience, motivation)
- Management (decisions)
- Method (work processes, organisational structures)
- Machine (workplace arrangement, machinery)
- Material (materials used, components)
- Market (customer behaviour, competition, job market)

The participants call out specific problem causes that are entered directly into the diagram. The causes, the elimination of which promises great success, can be determined in the next step using a multi-faceted prioritising question (see above).

2. Small Group Scenario

Application situations:
- Several topics are to be dealt with at the same time
- The group is too large for productive plenum work
- The participants only express themselves in a reserved manner in the plenum

Procedure:
First of all, agreement is reached on which topics can be dealt with simultaneously. Afterwards, the moderator presents the scenario for group work. Specific questions or headings for dealing with the topics are pre-formulated on the pinboard. The free spaces can be used to write down results. This scenario

provides the common denominator. The small groups are formed in such way that the participants allocate themselves to one of the topics according to interest, responsibility or skills. The groups withdraw to get to work (agree to a precise time plan!). In conclusion, they present their results in the plenum and put them up for discussion.

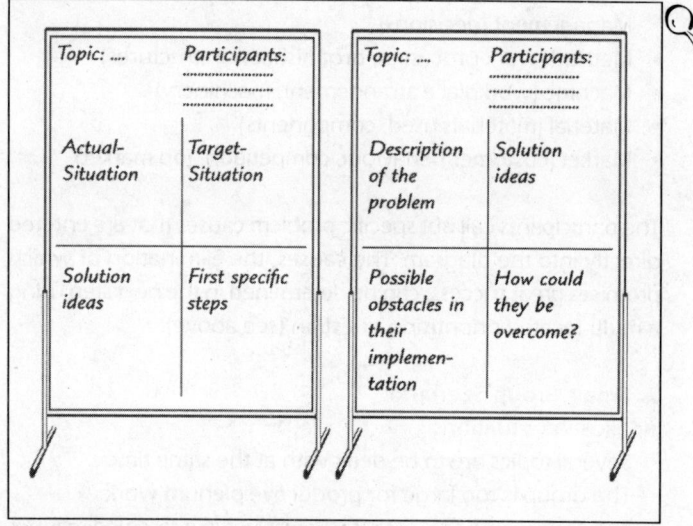

Ill. 14: Examples of small group scenarios

3. Brainstorming

Application situations:

- A broad number of the greatest variety of ideas is sought
- In the creative processes, the participants tend to fall into rash bickering or competitive behaviour

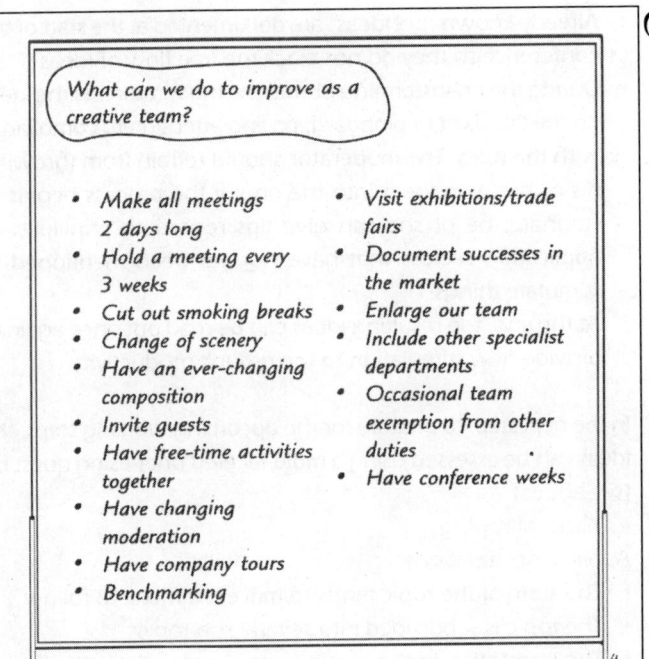

Ill. 15: Brainstorming

Procedure:

- The moderator announces the topic and presents the brainstorming rules:
  - Produce as many ideas as possible in the shortest possible amount of time (quantity takes precedence over quality here; only use catchphrases to describe the ideas)
  - Pick up on ideas from others and develop them further
  - Let your imagination run free
  - Refrain from criticising; do not rate or comment on ideas

- Already-known "pet ideas" are documented at the start of the conference so they do not block the free flow of ideas
- During the brainstorming phase, the moderator lists the ideas on the flip chart or pinboard, paying attention to compliance with the rules. The moderator should refrain from throwing his or her own ideas into the ring; if the process begins to stagnate, he or she can give tips regarding principles or application sectors that have not yet been mentioned to stimulate things.
- At the end, the resulting ideas can be read out once again to provide new stimulation to the group's productivity

In the next step, to prepare for the upcoming working steps, the ideas can be assessed using a multi-faceted prioritising question (see above).

4. Mind Mapping

Application situations:

- The state of the topic tends to make it difficult to follow
- The topic is subdivided into several sub-topics
- The interaction in the group moves associatively from topic to topic without any tangible result

Procedure:

- The moderator writes the topic in the middle of the flip chart or the pinboard
- He or she then draws branches and twigs from that point for the primary and secondary strands of the subject matter, writing keywords directly beside the branches (headings for allocation of the ideas)
- The participants call out their ideas and points of view and the moderator enters these directly into the "Mind Map"

Moderation Techniques and Visualisations

Later on, the Mind Map ideas can be evaluated using multi-faceted prioritising questions.

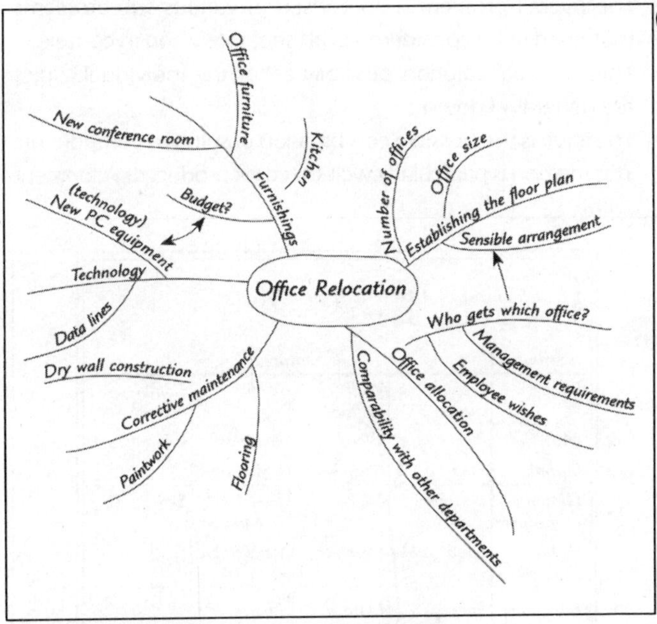

Ill. 16: Mind Map on the topic of office relocation

Tips for Mind Mapping

- *Make ideas obvious by using graphics and symbols*
- *Use different colours*
- *Create visual connections between the branches where links exist (e.g. lines, arrows)*
- *Amend your Mind Map whenever you think of something new*

5. Morphological Matrix

Application situations:

- The overall problem is comprised of various sub-problems that need to be considered both separately and in context
- The available solution possibilities for the individual topics are generally known
- The issue is the possible combination of solution components
- This method is particularly well-suited for product development

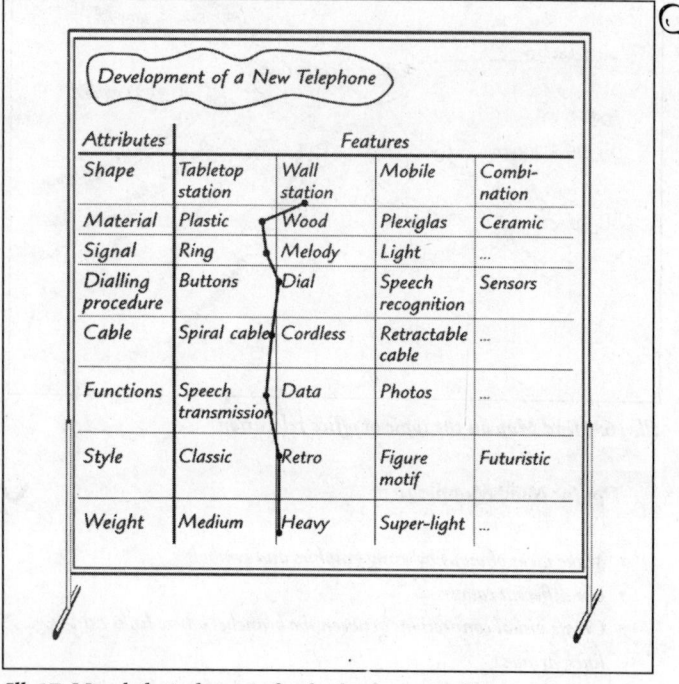

Ill. 17: Morphological matrix for the development of a new telephone

Moderation Techniques and Visualisations

Procedure:
- The group and the moderator formulate the question or the problem as precisely as possible.
- The moderator creates a visual of a matrix framework. As the group calls out, the moderator "fills in" the drawing according to the following scheme:
  - All of the parameters, i.e. all the structure elements designating the solution are listed vertically (sub-problems/topic components).
  - All conceivable solutions for the individual parameters are recorded horizontally (alternatives, variations).
- Combining the different solution variations reveals new solution possibilities for the overall problem. These can be connected to one another with lines.

The quality of the resulting solution combinations can be assessed together in the next step.

Tips for creating a morphological matrix

- *The parameters should be independent of one another so that the variations can be combined freely*
- *All important parameters should be documented*
- *Parameters that are not essential to the overall solution should be neglected. – For instance, a morphological matrix on automobiles does not have to contain the colour of the steering wheel as a parameter!*

Assessing Solutions – Decision Matrix

Application situations:
- Several solution alternatives are available for selection
- Several criteria influence the decision

- Not all of the determining factors are quantifiable
- Up to now, there has been a lack of clarity regarding the decision criteria and their priority

Decision for Cooperation Partner

Alternatives		Blitz GmbH		Ott GmbH	
Criteria	Priority	Grade	Priority	Grade	Priority
Business synergies	30%	4	1.2	6	1.8
Image	15%	6	0.9	4	0.6
Existing contacts	10%	6	0.6	3	0.3
Business forecast	25%	2	0.5	2	0.5
Corporate culture	20%	6	1.2	4	0.8
Sum		24	**4.4**	19	**4**

Ill. 18: Prioritised decision matrix

Procedure:
- The moderator draws a matrix framework
- The criteria that are important for the decision are entered along the vertical axis
- The solution alternatives are entered along the horizontal axis
- The group evaluates the extent to which the criteria are fulfilled in the various alternatives (e.g. 6 is the best value, 1 is the worst)

- The results are added together, visibly revealing which alternative receives the best mark

If the criteria are of varying significance, then the marks can also be prioritised. This can be done by applying percentage-prioritising of the criteria. The sum of the percentage shares should result in 100 %.

Agreeing Measures and Safeguarding Results – Measures Plan

Application situations:
- Resolutions, measures, responsibilities and deadlines should be documented

Procedure:
The measures chart is already prepared as a framework at the beginning of the conference, or the moderator creates it as soon as the first measure is agreed.

Measures				
No.	What?	Who?	By when?	Info to/Feedback
1	Explore cooperation possibilities with Blitz Inc.	Ms. Stern Mr. Paul	Oct. 14, 07	Report at the meeting on Oct. 21, 07
2	...	...	...	...

Ill. 19: Measures plan

Instructions for the columns:
- **No.:** Sequential number of the measure; this only serves to help maintain the overview and does not signify priority.
- **What:** The agreed activity is entered into the column.
- **Who:** The responsible person's name is entered here. For activities to be implemented by a number of persons, the entry should be the name of the main contact person.
- **By when:** The deadline for completing the measure is entered here.
- **Info to / Feedback:** The persons to be informed about the measure and when the group is to receive a status report are entered here.

Each measure is entered directly into the chart. At the end of the conference, everyone looks at the entire catalogue of measures: Has anything important been forgotten? Can individual measures be compiled sensibly into larger measures bundles? Is the scope of the discussed tasks realistic (Hygiene Check)? The measures plan is the core of the meeting results.

Closing – Meeting or Workshop Feedback

Application situations:
- The participants' satisfaction with the meeting is of great importance
- The participants are willing to talk openly about their personal perception of the meeting
- It is uncertain whether the assessment of the meeting will be the same by all the participants

Procedure:
- The moderator outlines the coordinate system with the dimensions "Factual Result" and "Process"

Moderation Techniques and Visualisations

- Each participant receives an adhesive dot with which to indicate their individual satisfaction on the chart (for instance, high satisfaction with the result and high satisfaction with the process – high satisfaction with the result and low satisfaction with the process ...)
- In conclusion, each participant gives a brief comment on their own evaluation of the meeting

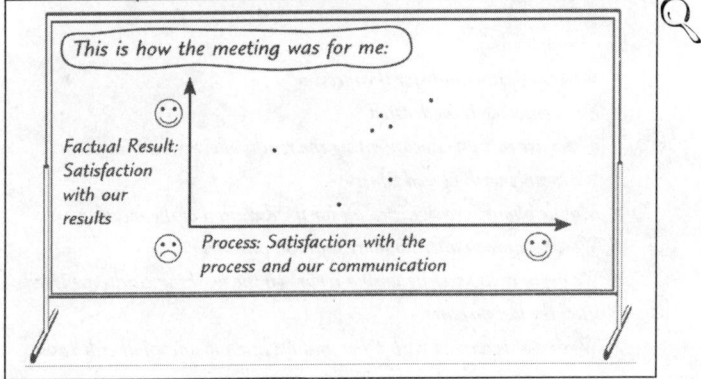

Ill. 20: Meeting Feedback

4.3 Rules for Meetings

Agree binding rules with your team! Rules make the standard of your meetings transparent and increase the satisfaction of the team members.

Many companies create binding meeting rules that are applicable for all internal conferences. Sometimes they are visibly displayed in the conference rooms as posters, and these rules are subsequently a firm component of the company culture. Here are a few tried-and-tested meeting rules as suggestions.

Rules for meetings

Preparation:
- The person responsible for the meeting distributes the agenda to the participants at least three days in advance
- There is a party responsible for each item on the agenda
- We prepare for the topics on the agenda

Execution:
- We arrive punctually for the meeting
- Every meeting is moderated
- There are minutes documenting the results of every meeting
- We comply with agreed times
- Mobile phones are switched off for the duration of the meeting
- We take a break after no more than 60 minutes
- We begin each meeting with a report on the working results achieved since the last meeting
- We do not interrupt each other and we listen to one another because every contribution is important
- We condense our thoughts so as to get to the point and keep our comments brief, ensuring that everyone has the chance to speak
- We are all responsible for reaching the aspired objectives
- If something is bothering us, we address it openly
- We do not allow any personal attacks
- The moderator has the permission and the obligation to make sure the discussion sticks to the topic
- Each meeting is concluded with a result consisting either of a decision or the agreement of a measure
- Each result will be documented immediately

Follow-Up:
- *Every participant receives the minutes of the meeting no later than three days after its conclusion*
- *We complete the tasks we have assumed during the meeting consistently and punctually*
- *When a task has been completed, the person responsible for the topic receives a brief report*
- *If a task cannot be completed, then the person who assumed it will endeavour to find a solution to enable the task to be completed after all. If this is not possible, then the person responsible for the topic must be informed*

Particularly in the case of meetings held in-house, there are often interruptions and disruptions that may seem harmless enough in and of themselves, but that can be a genuine irritation if they occur too frequently. For instance, an employee comes in and "just needs a signature" from one of the participants, or a participant is called out of the meeting to take a phone call. To offset this, some teams use the "100 km" rule: The only interruptions allowed are those that would be unavoidable if the meeting was taking place at a location 100 kilometres away from the company premises.

5 Roles and Posture of the Moderator

What is expected of the moderator and what is his or her role? – In practice, we generally find three types in the role of the director: The moderator is either a manager, a colleague of equal rank (and subsequently, if applicable, subordinate to the higher-ranking participants present) or an externally appointed Meeting Director.

5.1 A Manager as Moderator

This is generally the case. The manager meets with his or her team on a weekly basis, for example, or the board meets under the direction of the chief executive. The combination of the role of boss and moderator has its advantages, but also its disadvantages.

Resources:

- As a rule, the position of power automatically guarantees personal acceptance of the director by the participants
- Streamlined meeting direction is possible
- Usually a higher-ranking individual as the director has a high degree of factual knowledge and general knowledge of the organisation and the work-related environment. This simplifies a goal-oriented, effective procedure.

Limits and obstacles:

- Keeping the roles of boss and moderator separate is often not so easy. If the boss asserts his or her own position as the director, then it can sometimes be difficult to fall back into the role of the moderator
- A boss in the director's role can sometimes be overly dominant
- If conflicts surface, then the director is usually seen less as a moderator and more as a referee who is expected to make a judgement call

Roles and Posture of the Moderator

Recommendation:

As a boss in the role of director, always signal clearly when you are acting as either the moderator or the boss. For instance, you might stand whenever you are acting as the moderator and sit whenever you want to make factual or technical contributions to the discussion. Also, whenever you are heavily involved with a particular agenda item, you can delegate the role of director to another person for the duration of the related discussion.

5.2 A Team Colleague of Equal Rank as the Moderator

In many teams, the members are responsible for taking turns as the moderator of the team's meetings. This reinforces a balanced assumption of responsibility. Bosses benefit from this to the extent that they can concentrate more fully on observing the process and on their role as coach of the team. Additionally, having team members assume the demanding role of moderator represents an active contribution to personnel development.

Resources:
- Generally speaking, a colleague in the role of moderator invests effort into preparation in order to make a particularly good impression on the other colleagues and the boss.
- In the "appointed" role of director, a colleague usually acts in a manner that is attentive and cooperative.
- As a colleague who is familiar with the work from the ground up, the moderator knows "what is what" and subsequently pays attention to the practical relevance of the discussion contributions.
- Employee competence and motivation rise; regular rotation of the moderator role increases the willingness to assume responsibility throughout the entire team.

Individualism vs. Collectivism

What do you think is happening here?

An American manager working in Japan is particularly impressed by the performance of one of his team. At the next team meeting he praises this person in front of the group. The rest of the Japanese team look uneasy.

Japan is seen to be a highly collectivist culture — decisions are made by the group rather than by individuals. The Japanese are uneasy because one of the group has been singled out for attention. A better approach would be for the US manager to praise the work of the whole team.

Individualist cultures stress self-realisation whereas collectivist ones require that the individual fits into the group. The collectivist idea is illustrated by the Japanese saying "The nail that stands out must be hammered down." In individualist cultures people look after themselves and their immediate family, whereas in collectivist ones they look after a wider group in exchange for loyalty.

Collectivist cultures (e.g. South America, East Asia, West Africa) tend to have the following features:
- identity is based on the social network which you belong to
- communication is high context (cf. p. 33)
- employer-employee relationship is like a family link

Individualist cultures (e.g. USA, North-Western Europe, Australia) tend to have the following features:
- identity is based on the individual
- communication is low context (cf. p. 33)
- employer-employee relationship is based on a contract

(adapted from Hofstede, 1991, p. 67)

Roles and Posture of the Moderator

Limits and obstacles:
- In controversial group processes or personal conflicts, the colleague as moderator can often be overwhelmed because of a lack of distance to the problem and also a lack of training in guiding the team through troubled waters.
- The boss present at the meeting can sometimes tend to "rain on the parade" of the moderating employee in order to assert one of his or her favourite ideas.

Recommendation:
Make use of the opportunity as a manager to give your employees "on the job" training as moderators. Be attentive during the entire meeting so that when critical situations arise you can provide a safety net for the moderating employee, but intervene as little as possible. Allow the employee to gain experience and develop an individual moderation style.

As an employee, do not miss out on the chance to apply for the role of moderator if it is offered and take advantage of the opportunity to actively develop your professional skills.

5.3 An External Moderator to Guide the Process

Generally speaking, an external moderator is only called upon if there is good reason. Sometimes the aspired objectives simply cannot be achieved by the means available to the internal team. This is where an outside party as moderator comes in – perhaps a corporate consultant. But this person could also be a trained moderator from within the ranks of the company who normally has little contact with the team in question. Many larger companies in particular have in-house moderator pools. External

moderators are often requested in the following situations:
- Complex subjects must be addressed with professional methodical procedures
- The direction of a neutral person who is not involved in the technical and interpersonal dynamics of the team is desired
- There is a decided focus on dealing with conflicts
- External moderation is used as an introduction to a longer-term team development process

Resources:
- The moderator can help the team to acquire a view beyond "the end of its nose", so to speak, by using unaccustomed questioning and procedural methods.
- Given appropriate training, the external moderator, together with the group, can constructively work out complex technical procedures and controversial interpersonal dynamics.
- The external moderator can ease the burden of contentious situations: If the "flames" rise higher, then it is less risky if an external moderator "gets burned" than if an insider is damaged.

Limits and obstacles:
- As a rule, an external moderator does not possess any deep-rooted expertise in the field of the work topic of the team, meaning extensive advance briefing is required. But even then, the moderator will still have little detailed specialised knowledge.
- To work intensively, the moderator needs a certain amount of "warm-up" time with the team, generally requiring at least half a day.

- Sometimes too much is expected of the moderator: His or her job is to repair conflicts that have emerged in some cases over the course of years in only a few hours using "tricks and techniques". Anyone appointing (and accepting) such assignments can only lose.

Recommendations:

Many teams are reluctant to engage external moderators, since this costs more time and money. In addition, it is a natural tendency to want to avoid making the impression that one can not handle one's own problems alone. Sometimes this means that the difficulties are festering in the background for so long that even an experienced moderator is unable to steer the situation in a more positive direction. For this reason, it is recommended that external moderation is called upon before things have gone too far. For moderators, it is recommended that they precisely clarify the situation of the team and the objective of the meeting in advance, and only accept appointments that can be brought to a successful conclusion.

5.4 The Neutral, Appreciative Posture of the Moderator

The methodological skills enable the moderator to assist the group process. The moderator's knowledge and experience are made available to the group. He or she supports the communication within the group so that it is able to process relevant solutions in a structured way and the group members are able to arrange their relationships with one another in a positive manner. Neutrality, appreciative respect towards the participants, refraining from making personal assessments and great personal integrity are the distinguishing characteristics of a good moderator. He understands that disruptions and conflicts represent important signals in the working process for which the moderator provides methods so that they can be worked out constructively. The moderator's behaviour is oriented along the guidelines outlined below.

Fundamental principles for moderators

- *Only moderate events where you have done the preparation yourself*
- *Do not permit individuals to manipulate the meeting for their own purposes*
- *Insist on professional execution and documentation*
- *Refrain from the urge to provide the solution to problems yourself, and arouse the potential of the participants instead*
- *Do not allow persons to be degraded*
- *Make sure the work process is transparent*
- *Make sure that consensus can be seen as consensus and that dissent is well-founded*
- *Do not struggle against the group (keep your opinion to yourself, trust the process and the participants, do not egg the group on)*
- *Do not stand in judgement over statements made by participants*
- *Make your appearance as emotionally neutral as possible*

6 Guiding the Group Process

It is the job of the moderator to exercise a positive influence on the dynamics of the emotions and the interpersonal relationships in the team. We will address this issue in this chapter.

6.1 Four Levels of Group Communication

It is helpful for you as a moderator to precisely register the processes and dynamics that are simultaneously at work in meetings. You can observe four levels of dynamics in particular:

Content
Discussion of topics and objectives, professional competence, rational argumentation
Procedure
Agreements, methodology, bylaws, formal roles, guiding the course of the meeting
Relationships
Closeness – distance, sympathy – antipathy, the group climate, informal roles/power
Individuals
Personal values, visions, needs, skills, motives, experiences

Ill. 21: Group communication levels (based on Rosenkranz)

First Level: Content

This level is the most accessible. The issue here consists of the factual topics and objectives to be attained. As such, this level determines the tenor of things, since the primary purpose of meetings is to get factual topics moving: A project should be finished on time, a management planning measure needs working out, and so on.

However, at times focusing solely on the factual topic can lead to paying too little attention to other processes; for instance, when the group becomes so immersed in a discussion that, ultimately, the time designated for important topics is insufficient, or when critical fact-related comments lead to an aggressive atmosphere in the group. At such points, discourse of a purely content-relevant nature reaches its limits; the process and relationship level (see below) then moves centre-stage.

> **You can positively influence group processes at the content level when you ...**

- *adequately familiarise yourself with the content*
- *communicate understandably*
- *ask about important facts*
- *promote the communication of the participants with one another*
- *exercise Active Listening*
- *introduce preliminary compilations*
- *use visualisation possibilities*
- *formulate objectives and agreements clearly*
- *make sure the documentation of the results is conducted properly*

Second Level: The Procedure

This level relates to the structure of the meeting. Is there an agenda as a common thread? What topics are to be dealt with in what order? What happens with the results? Who decides what?

The Meeting Director is responsible for the orderly running of the meeting and the transparency of the procedures. He or she ensures clarity and leads the team through the programme.

> **You can constructively guide group processes at the procedure level when you ...**

- *create clarity with the team regarding the agenda*
- *keep an eye on the timeframes*
- *keep the common thread in view from time to time*
- *consistently ensure that the rules are complied with*
- *regularly request feedback on the acceptance of the procedures; ask whether the group is still on the right track*
- *obtain consensus about how to proceed in the event of disruptions*
- *slow down processes if necessary; take the time to obtain important clarifications*
- *make sure that the agreement of tasks and assignments is understood to be binding*

Third Level: Relationships

Even in meetings focused on factual matters, we still enter into a relationship with the other participants. Some team members have known each other for a long time and have great empathy for one another. Others already enter the meeting arena as opponents; the meeting becomes the staging ground for their conflicts. And still others are meeting for the first time and are carefully looking for their place among the other participants. A fundamental principle of interpersonal communication is:

The relationship level characterises the content level. Human beings are frequently guided to a far greater extent by sympathy and antipathy than by rational thought. Negative emotions can significantly disrupt the working process, sometimes without those affected even recognising it. The conflict smoulders and suddenly cannot be reigned in by factual discussion. The communication in groups can often be accurately described with the assistance of the Iceberg Metaphor:

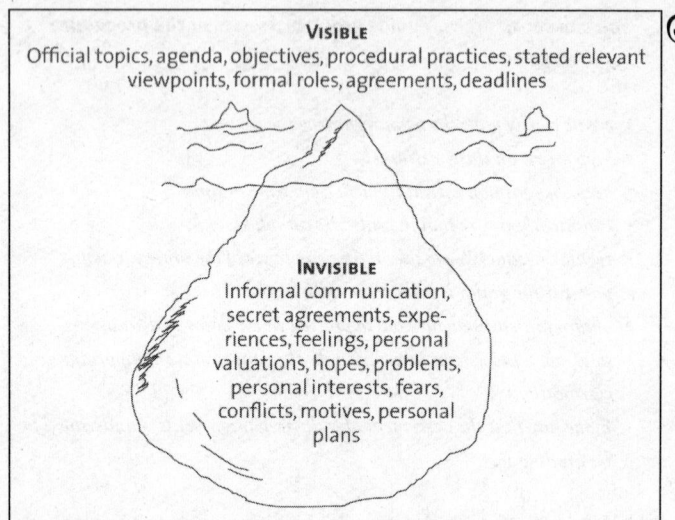

Ill. 22: The Iceberg Model of group communication

Above the surface of the water – i.e. accessible to the conscious mind – is where the work on tangible matters takes place; information is provided, knowledge is absorbed, discussion is conducted (10 % of the energy). But below the surface, movement is caused by attraction and repulsion, hopes and fears, injuries and conflicts (90 % of the energy).

A positive relationship climate in a meeting based on appreciation makes working at the procedural level easy, because less energy is needed for protection against attacks or coming to terms with insults that have been suffered. This leaves all the energy available for reaching the objectives together.

The body is the medium for all our emotions and relationships. *"Our hair is standing on end"*, we say, or *"we feel attracted to someone"* or perhaps *"repelled by someone"*. Handling things at the relationship level means above all having a sensitive perception of body language signals and also being aware of the impression one's own body language makes as a moderator.

> **You can positively influence group processes at the relationship level when you ...**

- *ensure a framework that is free of stress and is communication-friendly*
- *provide sufficient space for the participants to get acquainted with one another when necessary*
- *show all of the participants your appreciation*
- *provide a sense of security through clear, attentive moderation*
- *promote cooperation between the participants*
- *allow distance*
- *allow conflicts without taking sides*
- *pay attention to the body language signals of the participants – above all, those that signal uneasiness or discord*
- *pay attention to your own body language (warning) signals*
- *make sure to speak with a relaxed voice and leave enough pauses when speaking*
- *make it easier to express feelings using appropriate methods when needed (cf. Part B, Chapters 2.8, 4.2)*
- *are a reliable, trustworthy dialogue partner*

Fourth Level: Individuals

When we appear in a conference room, we always carry with us a backpack loaded with all of the experiences we have collected throughout our lives. Why did we choose a particular profession? What do we seek to achieve in our professional lives? Why do we find an affinity with some group members, while finding none at all with others? The answers to these types of questions can often be found deep within our personalities and our individual development.

Differences between group members are demonstrated in large part in relation to ...
- values and attitudes
- personal objectives
- motivation
- working style
- needs
- talents and skills
- self-confidence

> Respecting and appreciating all of the participants in their differences is the most important fundamental basis of good moderation.

On this basis, your interventions will find acceptance, even in situations that are difficult.

Goal-orientation and rules for the process create a framework that each person should comply with. Nonetheless, the level of the personalities of each of the participants plays a big role in every meeting. Sometimes behaviour that initially seemed to make no sense becomes crystal clear with hindsight. For example, an employee who normally is a go-getter is suddenly taking a back seat in assuming project tasks; later we learn that the person in question had already been planning to change jobs at that point in time.

It is often the skills of the moderator in allowing differences to occur within a meeting and even encouraging them that decide the extent to which the participants respect one another and come together as a group.

Guiding the Group Process

> **You can positively influence group processes at the level of individual needs when you ...**

- *create an atmosphere in which it is possible to express personal needs and (differing) views*
- *allow distance and allow participants (and yourself) the right to set boundaries for themselves*
- *ensure that, whatever the circumstances, none of the participants has to lose face*

Without a doubt, it is virtually impossible to consciously direct a meeting all the time at all four of the communication levels set out above. Moreover, the moderator undertakes many direction processes unconsciously. But the moderator can direct his or her attention to whether individual levels are receiving too little attention during the course of a meeting, resulting in irritations about the overall process.

One's own perception and requested feedback from the participants can help to recognise whether the participants ...
- are adequately focused on the content
- are finding the meeting sufficiently objective-oriented and structured
- have enough opportunity for exchanging views and nurturing relationships
- consider their needs as being appropriately looked after

Incidentally, meetings normally develop a healthy dynamic of their own, which should not be hindered through excessive direction.

Depending on the situation, individual levels of communication are particularly active. For instance, at the start the first priority is to provide clarifications on the agenda at the procedure level, while later in the course of a meeting that is running productively, one can concentrate fully on relevant content.

6.2 Moderation as Team Development
Workgroups and teams experience typical development phases. This results in various demands on the moderator.

Phases of Team Development

In practice, it can be observed that teams often go through certain typical phases in the development of their working capabilities. These phases are more easily noted by their designations as Forming, Storming, Norming and Performing.

- Forming: The team members explore the terrain with a certain degree of caution or excited anticipation. Their dealings with one another are notably courteous. Each person is looking for their place in the team.
- Storming: Now the issue is establishing the "pecking order" in the group. Dominant members form crystallisation points for emerging sub-groups. The role and strength of the director are also tested. A number of subliminal conflicts are perceptible, often resulting in some degree of neglect of the work on the actual relevant subject matter in this phase.
- Norming: The various needs are discussed openly; rules are established: Who may do what? What do we expect of each other? These clarifications ease the dealings with one another. The team becomes more productive.
- Performing: The team has found itself. It utilises its potentials and works towards its objectives. Dealings with one another are unconstrained. Personal contacts have emerged within the group. The energy of the team is very appealing for outsiders.

The phases of team development are often described as a wheel, since the cycle of phases is passed through again with every change in the constellation of the team. The phases of team development do not occur on a linear basis; some things happen simultaneously: While some are still seeking their role and causing or experiencing friction with other team members, others have already found a way to make effective contributions.

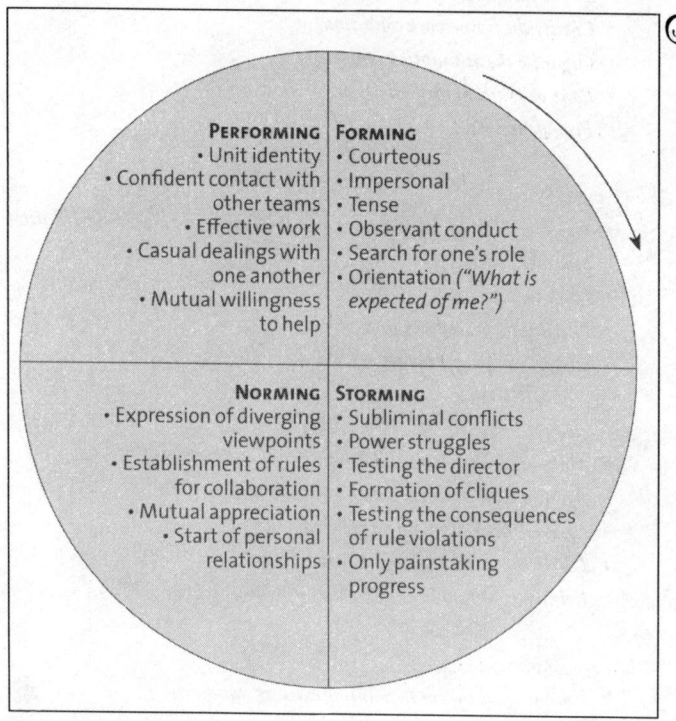

Ill. 23: The wheel of team development

Help from the Moderator

As a moderator, you should look closely at what interventions are helpful for the team's growth process.

> **Intervention tips for the four team development phases**

Forming:
- *Enable the participants to become acquainted with one another*
- *Clarify the framework conditions*
- *Organise the assumption of duties*
- *Positive praise of the first actions of the team*
- *Provide security*

Storming:
- *Welcome differences of opinion and conflicts as important clarification processes*
- *Mediate conflicts*
- *Nip unfair procedures in the bud*
- *Clarify working processes*

Norming:
- *Motivate the team to establish rules*
- *Agree on objectives for which everyone is responsible*
- *Promote discussions and open feedback*
- *Direct the team's view outwards*
- *Reinforce mutual trust and the assumption of responsibility*

Performing:
- *Encourage the team to examine existing standards*
- *Promote team self-supervision*
- *Tone down the directorship role – establishment of rotating moderation*

- *Make successes visible*
- *Find new, challenging visions and objectives*
- *Promote a feedback culture and openness to new influences*

With many tasks, the team performance far exceeds the sum of the possible individual performances of the participants. Often enough, the emerging team begins to believe that what it has now started will continue unabated indefinitely.

But teams are subject to change, because the environment and the personal needs of the participants change over time. The intoxicating feeling of strength that teams sometimes develop also conceals a certain degree of risk. The focus dwindles; new areas of conflict emerge virtually unnoticed within the group. External dynamics of change are not recognised early enough. As the director, view each meeting as a new beginning; you can contribute in this way to the process of keeping the team "young".

7 Dealing with Challenging Behaviour

Moderators receive a myriad of recommendations on how to deal with various participant "types". These include classifying people in groups, such as *"The Speechmaker"*, *"The Quiet One"*, *"The Aggressive One"* or even *"The Unruly One"*. These stark, deprecating classifications often make it more rather than less difficult for the moderator to deal with varying types of participant behaviour.

So instead, here are a few tips for handling certain typical behavioural patterns that often prove challenging, because if someone becomes aggressive during a meeting, for instance, it does not necessarily mean that this is an overly aggressive person; it could signify that the person in question is currently under stress or was irritated by what was just said or done. And the person who is (still) quietly participating in the meeting may well be sizing up the situation before becoming actively involved. Be aware that conduct depends above all on the situation, and as such is flexible and subject to influence.

Tips for dealing with challenging behaviour

Reservation and reticence:
- *Tolerate, do not immediately intervene*
- *Make eye contact repeatedly and do not "forget" the reserved participant*
- *Look for "linkage points" to the work area of the reserved person during the course of the meeting and ask questions about their personal experience*
- *If the entire group is reserved, introduce partner and group work to "ease the freeze" among the participants*

Dealing with Challenging Behaviour

Dominant behaviour:
- *Permit the person in question to articulate suggestions*
- *Praise ideas and active participation*
- *Ask questions or let the group ask questions*
- *Let the group make comments*
- *As the director, do not build up any rivalries and do not be easily impressed*
- *When the respective person's contribution is concluded, thank them for their contribution and go forward with the moderation*

Speechmaking, overly long comments:
- *Maintain an atmosphere of appreciation*
- *Praise the multitude of aspects mentioned*
- *Block tactfully (see all of Chapter 2.7 in Part B)*
- *At the appropriate opportunity, make a general request for brief contributions*

Aggressive behaviour:
- *Remain calm*
- *Acknowledge that the great emotional commitment of the person in question is recognised – use temperate language*
- *In cases of general, unspecific agitation: If necessary, ask where or at what person the irritation is directed*

Moaning, continuous criticism, "killer phrases":
- *Ask the group to neutrally analyse the content of the criticism*
- *Ask the person or persons in question what the real reason is for the dissatisfaction ...*
- *In conclusion, clarify with the group whether working out the dissatisfaction is an issue that belongs in the meeting or requires another forum*

Personal attacks and abuse:
- Confront the procedure directly and unmistakably (remain fair in doing so); make it clear that such behaviour will not be accepted

Wisecracks, clowning:
- Enjoy the relaxed conduct as long as it stays within reasonable limits – praise positive effects
- If it becomes obvious that the participants view the conduct as a disruption, ask the person in question to state his or her position on the relevant topical matter – afterwards let the group comment.
- In case of a massive disruption of the group, ask the group tactfully to comment on the conduct
- If necessary, seek out a discussion in private with the person in question

8 Conflict Clarification

As a moderator, you should recognise the first signs of conflict early on. If grave personal insults hang in the air, it is usually difficult to find a way back to an unprejudiced, constructive collaboration. And the reason for this is simple: Even if the topic has been cleared up, the negative emotional aftertaste of what happened has left an impression in us that can scarcely be dissolved again with intellectual processes. It is therefore preferable in many cases to prevent the conflict than to deal with it.

8.1 Signs of Conflict Dynamics – The Progression of Conflicts

It is all well and good that discussions sometimes heat up in meetings. After all, everyone is trying to achieve something: Various participants are trying to obtain access to the same scarce resources, inherently competing objectives are to be reached simultaneously, etc. But what is even more decisive than the topic representing the source of the controversy is the manner in which it is dealt with. Here are a few warning signs that you should observe as a moderator:

Active conflict conduct
- Continuous drawn out discussion contributions from individual participants
- Interrupting others while they are talking
- Incessant repetition of the same arguments
- Bringing up old stories
- Overall criticism, generalisations (*"always"*, *"never"*)
- Personal attacks, accusations of incompetence
- Irony, cynicism

- Concealed and open threats ("*Oh, you'll see ...*")
- Deeds (storming out of the room, slamming doors)

Passive Conflict Conduct
- Withdrawal from the communication, disinterest
- Blocking of decisions, intransigence,
- Subservience, distanced politeness, exaggerated friendliness

In the case of active conflict conduct, you should immediately intervene. With passive behaviour, you can "test the wind" by cautiously asking about the reason for the unusual behaviour – in the end, it is up to the person you suspect of being more withdrawn whether he or she wants to specify the nature of the conflict openly in the group. The basic principle is not to be pushy!

You should not try to be the referee without being asked to do so. You have a clear mandate at the point when the conflict partners ask you to mediate the conflict – and to do so, you need the request from both conflict parties.

Another situation where you actually must intervene is when you, as a manager, recognise a conflict between two employees who are answerable to you that they themselves cannot resolve and that is having an overall detrimental effect on the success of the work or the working environment.

Typical Conflict Progressions
If conflict situations are not steered onto a constructive path, then they often take the following course:

1. Latent conflict
- Individuals or everyone senses displeasure without articulating it openly
- Discussions become more temperamental

Conflict Clarification

2. Open conflict
- The "line has been crossed": Internal or external causes (for example, unfulfilled expectations or instructions from "upstairs") have brought the conflict to a head
- Presented arguments are not granted credibility (anymore); accusations of self-interest and tactical behaviour emerge
- The conflict parties are increasingly emotionalised
- The respective conflict styles typical of the parties appear:
    - Battling
    - Submitting
    - Avoiding the other, withdrawing
    - Agreeing to compromises, "horse-trading"
    - Constructive work on the issue, searching for solutions to the problem

3. Escalation
- Anger and indignation emerge
- Allies are sought
- Words are followed by deeds
- Logic is forgone in favour of irrational actions

4. Hardening
- One party has won or a stalemate has emerged
- The "hot" conflict has now transformed into a "cold" conflict
- The two avoid one another instead of cooperating
- The potential for conflict remains; it can erupt again at the next best opportunity

Even the very style of dealing constructively with a conflict can clear up the situation on a long-term basis. The opportunities for a solution to the conflict are at their greatest when it has not yet boiled over into attacks, and also when the phase of positions hardening has not been reached.

8.2 Active Conflict Mediation

On the one hand, the moderator's contribution to the constructive settlement of conflicts consists of assisting in their de-escalation: Reasonable solutions are only possible when the parties begin talking to one another again. On the other hand, the moderator can help to come up with a satisfactory solution for everyone by implementing a problem-solving procedure (see Part B, Chapter 3.1). In conclusion, a few tips for mediating conflicts have been compiled here:

Tips for conflict mediation

- *Examine whether you are suitable as a conflict moderator. (Criteria: The moderator may not be personally involved in the conflict and should have been given a mandate to direct the process by both parties)*
- *Ensure a framework with the least possible amount of stress, and set aside sufficient time for the negotiations*
- *Show both parties your appreciation*
- *Ensure compliance with the rules*
  - *Both parties are equal*
  - *Both parties may say what they have to say without being interrupted*
  - *Problems should be addressed openly and directly*
  - *Have conduct, facts, views and experiences described in specific terms; do not permit any accusations and reproaches*
- *Encourage the parties to articulate their deeper lying interests*
- *Shed light on commonalities before addressing the areas where the viewpoints split*

- *Start with easy points that can be resolved quickly*
- *Emotions can be expressed openly – encourage "I-statements"*
- *Promote the communication of the conflicting parties with one another; ask them to put themselves in the position of the other*

Conflict Clarification

- *Intervene immediately and unmistakably when violations of the rules occur*
- *Reduce your direction **if you notice that the parties are entering into a constructive dialogue***
- ***Remain** neutral and patient*
- *Document the results*

- *No result should be granted final approval before all of the topics have been aired*
- ***Should new facts emerge that cannot be allocated immediately or if the exchange is lacking the necessary impulse, then call for a** pause for consideration **and agree to a new appointment for renewal of the discussion***
- *Agree on rules that will help to prevent re-emergence of the conflict*

Part C Follow-Up

The quality of a meeting is demonstrated above all in the implementation of its results. Binding, well-structured minutes are a prerequisite for this.

1 The Minutes

The minutes fulfil a variety of functions:
- Documentation of decisions and ideas
- Planning basis for subsequent activities
- Information basis for persons not attending the meeting
- Impetus for the next meeting

In practice, one usually finds two types of minutes:
- Resolution minutes: This variation is used most frequently. It only documents results and decisions.
- Session minutes: This version documents results and decisions in addition to containing a condensed summary of the course of the discussion.

1.1 The Role of the Minutes Taker

The minutes taker must be capable of keeping up with the train of thought within the meeting and accurately recording the results. If resolutions are formulated in an unclear manner, it is important that he or she immediately asks for clarification and, if in doubt, takes dictation of the exact reading.

If controversial topics have been addressed in the meeting or if the minutes taker has little experience, it is recommended that the party calling the meeting reviews the minutes before they are sent to the participants.

The question regarding who is to take the minutes should be resolved no later than at the start of the meeting, so that decisions do not have to be reconstructed from memory.

There are various possibilities for determining the responsibility for the minutes:
- Rotating responsibility for the minutes
- There is a person whose role in the particular meeting is to take the minutes – for example, an assistant
- Someone takes the minutes who always does it well and who also has no objection to recording the results

The results of the meeting are often also recorded by the moderator, for instance on a flip chart. The advantage of this is that everyone can see the documentation of the results and immediately draw attention to any discrepancies.

1.2 Components of the Minutes

Integral components of the minutes are:
- The date and location of the meeting, participants
- Distribution list ("To:")
- Topics / Agenda items addressed
- Resolutions, assignments with responsible parties
- Date of the next meeting, if necessary
- Host, Meeting Director and minutes taker

When needed, additional documents can be added to the minutes for a better understanding of the meeting:
- Preparation documents, invitation and agenda
- List of participants
- Copies of presentations and speeches

1.3 Minutes Standard and Form

Many organisations use standard forms for their minutes. This enables new teams to benefit from organisational knowledge and also allows the documentation to be better understood and processed further by other parties involved. This is most important when project work plays a large role in the organisation. With a standard like this it is important to select the least bureaucratic form possible (see Ill. 24).

1.4 Photo Minutes

These days, session minutes are often produced as photo minutes containing all of the visualisations created during the meeting, as well as the measures plan.

Photo minutes provide three primary benefits:
- They save time: Photographing the charts is less work than actually writing the minutes
- Visualisation already makes all of the results visible for everyone during the course of the meeting
- All contributors can easily find the comments they made personally in the photo minutes

Digital cameras allow us today to almost effortlessly photograph the presented sheets and process them further on a PC.

The Minutes

MINUTES					
Topic:					
Location:		Company, city, address, bulding, room			
Date:		Date, time			
Participants:			To:		
....			....		
....			....		
....			....		
....			....		

RESULTS:

Cons. No.	Type:*	Keyword	Result/Resolution – Explaination	Reposible Party	Planned Deadline

*Result type: A = Assignment, Rs = Resolution,
R = Recommendation, S = Statement

Attachments/Appendixes:	Document designations
Next meeting:	Date, time, locations

Meeting dirctor:
Host:
Minutes Taker:

Distributed by:	Date, name of sender

Ill. 24: Example of a minutes form

2 Supporting Implementation

Anyone familiar with the day-to-day of project and team work knows that in many cases, implementing meeting results frequently requires active support. Agreed tasks often have to be taken care of outside the framework of the daily business, making them more susceptible to slipping down the priority list. As the person responsible for the team, this is a special challenge for you, because the success of your team will be measured by the quality of its implementation.

Tips for supporting implementation

- *After a certain period of time, call the participants and show interest*
- *Have the participants provide you with intermediate reports*
- *Report the initial implementation results and successes to the participants*
- *Ask about the progress of implementation from time to time*
- *Start subsequent meetings with a follow-up of the minutes from the previous meeting*

3 Personal Follow-Up Work of the Moderator

As a moderator, you should take some time after every meeting to review its progress and results for yourself. Your personal follow-up work can provide you with important findings and ideas for subsequent meetings. Here are some sample questions to get you going:

- Factual follow-up work:
  - Have we reached our objectives? If not, why not?
  - Were we able to work on all the topics? If not, what happens now to those topics we did not address?
  - Were new topics added?
  - Did I take on assignments myself? (Completion planning)
- Process-related follow-up work:
  - Were the methods used appropriate?
  - Was the preparation / the script right?
  - Did we use our time well?
  - Were the roles clearly defined?
  - Did the discussion have a good balance between structure and vitality?
  - Did everyone comply with the rules? Did I pay enough attention to compliance with the rules?
  - Are our agreements binding?
- Climate-related follow-up work:
  - How did I interpret the mood during the meeting?
  - Were all participants able to make a sufficient contribution?
  - Did we handle disruptions appropriately?
  - Was I able to emanate calm and security?

- Organisational follow-up work:
  - Were the agenda and the invitation correct?
  - Were the room and the media okay?
  - Are preparation and distribution of the minutes being dealt with?

Questionnaire: Assessment of Our Meetings Practice

As the person responsible for the team, you should continuously keep a watchful eye on the practice of your meetings in order to maintain the efficiency of your team and to recognise early on when misunderstandings begin to creep into your meetings. Regular flashlight rounds (cf. Part B, Chapter 2.8) and visualised meeting feedback rounds are a great help with this. Approximately once annually, you should take the time to talk comprehensively within the team about your meetings practice. With the aid of the questionnaire presented here, you and your team members can evaluate the current status of your meetings: It is of course important that everyone participates voluntarily.

Objectives:
- Discovering the strengths and weaknesses of how the meetings are conducted
- Creating the basis for the agreement on specific measures

Duration: Approximately two hours, including the assessment

Material:
- A questionnaire, notepad and pen for each participant (the publisher grants you permission to reproduce this questionnaire for internal, non-commercial use)
- Flip chart or pinboard with several sheets of paper, felt tip markers, adhesive dots

Course of the Meeting:

1. The participants individually tick off to what extent the statements contained in the questionnaire are true in their opinion.
2. Afterwards, they transfer their appraisals using adhesive dots onto the prepared flip chart or pinboard sheets, which display the statements in the identical form that they are contained in the questionnaire.
3. The team leader and the team evaluate the result together; after taking an overall look at the result, proceed then at best by going through each question individually. Evaluation aides:
   - *"Are we satisfied with the result?"*
   - "Do our appraisals of the individual questions concur, or are there 'blips'?" ("What are the reasons for this?")
   - "What do we want to achieve on the respective issue?"
   - *"What measures seem reasonable to us for accomplishing this?"*

Meetings Practice Questionnaire

No. Statement	Always true	Usually true	Seldom true	False
PREPARATION AND ORGANISATION:				
1. I understand the objectives of our meetings.	❏	❏	❏	❏
2. Meeting objectives are formulated so that everyone understands them.	❏	❏	❏	❏

3. Our meetings take place at the right intervals: Not too frequently and not too seldomly.	☐	☐	☐	☐
4. Our meeting agendas are formulated transparently.	☐	☐	☐	☐
5. I receive all the information early enough to prepare for the meetings.	☐	☐	☐	☐
6. The framework conditions of our meetings promote productive work (e.g. room, media, seating arrangement).	☐	☐	☐	☐
7. The time and duration of our meetings are chosen well.	☐	☐	☐	☐
8. In our team, all of the resources are available for us to be able to competently discuss the topics at hand.	☐	☐	☐	☐
9. External specialists are invited at the precise time that we need them to help resolve existing problems.	☐	☐	☐	☐

EXECUTION:

10. All team members feel free to state their views openly.	☐	☐	☐	☐
11. The team members' opportunities to speak are balanced.	☐	☐	☐	☐
12. We listen to one another attentively.	☐	☐	☐	☐

Personal Follow-Up Work of the Moderator

13. New ideas are taken on board positively by the team and we deal with innovative impulses constructively.	❏	❏	❏	❏
15. We discuss matters critically and controversially so that the best solutions rise to the top in the end.	❏	❏	❏	❏
16. Our methods are appropriate for our topics and objectives.	❏	❏	❏	❏
17. Decisions are made in a manner that is transparent and appropriate.	❏	❏	❏	❏
18. The agreements that we make are formulated in a way that is comprehensible and binding.	❏	❏	❏	❏
19. The working environment is positive and motivating.	❏	❏	❏	❏
20. We have found a good way of dealing with disruptions and conflicts.	❏	❏	❏	❏
21. We have set up enough rules to be able to arrange our meetings effectively.	❏	❏	❏	❏
22. We comply with our rules.	❏	❏	❏	❏
23. We have found a good balance between "Moderation by the Director" and "Self-Supervision by the Team".	❏	❏	❏	❏
24. With us, moderation is conducted in such a way that all information and factual assessments receive a fair hearing.	❏	❏	❏	❏

25. The moderation helps us to achieve our meeting objectives more quickly.	☐	☐	☐	☐
26. The moderation helps us to speak about our sensibilities and feelings.	☐	☐	☐	☐
27. It is good to have a moderator in our ranks who brings us back on track when discussions heat up.	☐	☐	☐	☐
28. We spend enough time talking about how to better arrange our meetings.	☐	☐	☐	☐
Follow-Up Work: 29. Our minutes contain all the important matters from the meeting.	☐	☐	☐	☐
30. We adequately ensure that our meeting results are implemented.	☐	☐	☐	☐
31. We receive enough feedback on the results of our work together.	☐	☐	☐	☐

Bibliography

- **Antons, K.:** Praxis der Gruppendynamik. Übungen und Techniken. **8. Auflage. Göttingen u. a. 2000.**
- **Barker, A.:** How to Manage Meetings. **London 2002.**
- **Doppler, K., Lauterburg, C.:** Change Management. Den Unternehmenswandel gestalten. **2. Auflage. Frankfurt/M., New York 1994.**
- **Francis, D. u. Young, D.:** Mehr Erfolg im Team. Ein Trainingsprogramm mit 46 Übungen zur Verbesserung der Leistungsfähigkeit in Arbeitsgruppen. **5. Auflage. Hamburg 1998.**
- **Gibson, R.:** Intercultural Business Communication. **Berlin 2000.**
- **Hall, E.:** Beyond Culture. **New York 1976**
- **Hofstede, G.:** Cultures and organizations. **London 1991.**
- **Klebert, K. u. a.:** ModerationsMethode. Das Standardwerk. **Hamburg 2002.**
- Manage meetings positively. **London 2006.**
- **Rosenkranz, H.:** Von der Familie zur Gruppe zum Team. Familien- und gruppendynamische Modelle zur Teamentwicklung. **2. Auflage. Paderborn 1994.**